NATIONAL ACADEMIES

Sciences
Engineering
Medicine

NATIONAL
ACADEMIES
PRESS
Washington, DC

T0285374

Future State of Smallpox Medical Countermeasures

Lawrence O. Gostin, Lisa Brown, Shalini Singaravelu,
and Matthew Masiello, *Editors*

Committee on the Current State of Research,
Development, and Stockpiling of Smallpox Medical
Countermeasures

Board on Health Sciences Policy

Board on Global Health

Health and Medicine Division

Board on Life Sciences

Division on Earth and Life Studies

Consensus Study Report

NATIONAL ACADEMIES PRESS 500 Fifth Street, NW Washington, DC 20001

This activity was supported by contracts between the National Academy of Sciences and the Administration for Strategic Preparedness and Response (75A50121C00061). Any opinions, findings, conclusions, or recommendations expressed in this publication do not necessarily reflect the views of any organization or agency that provided support for the project.

International Standard Book Number-13: 978-0-309-71737-3
International Standard Book Number-10: 0-309-71737-x
Digital Object Identifier: https://doi.org/10.17226/27652
Library of Congress Control Number: 2024937873

This publication is available from the National Academies Press, 500 Fifth Street, NW, Keck 360, Washington, DC 20001; (800) 624-6242 or (202) 334-3313; http://www.nap.edu.

Suggested citation: National Academies of Sciences, Engineering, and Medicine. 2024. *Future state of smallpox medical countermeasures*. Washington, DC: The National Academies Press. https://doi.org/10.17226/27652.

The **National Academy of Sciences** was established in 1863 by an Act of Congress, signed by President Lincoln, as a private, nongovernmental institution to advise the nation on issues related to science and technology. Members are elected by their peers for outstanding contributions to research. Dr. Marcia McNutt is president.

The **National Academy of Engineering** was established in 1964 under the charter of the National Academy of Sciences to bring the practices of engineering to advising the nation. Members are elected by their peers for extraordinary contributions to engineering. Dr. John L. Anderson is president.

The **National Academy of Medicine** (formerly the Institute of Medicine) was established in 1970 under the charter of the National Academy of Sciences to advise the nation on medical and health issues. Members are elected by their peers for distinguished contributions to medicine and health. Dr. Victor J. Dzau is president.

The three Academies work together as the **National Academies of Sciences, Engineering, and Medicine** to provide independent, objective analysis and advice to the nation and conduct other activities to solve complex problems and inform public policy decisions. The National Academies also encourage education and research, recognize outstanding contributions to knowledge, and increase public understanding in matters of science, engineering, and medicine.

Learn more about the National Academies of Sciences, Engineering, and Medicine at **www.nationalacademies.org**.

v

MATTHEW WYNIA, Director, Center for Bioethics and Humanities, University of Colorado

ZHILONG YANG, Associate Professor, Department of Veterinary Pathobiology, School of Veterinary Medicine & Biomedical Sciences, Texas A&M University

Study Staff

LISA BROWN, Study Director
SHALINI SINGARAVELU, Program Officer
MATTHEW MASIELLO, Associate Program Officer
MARGARET McCARTHY, Research Associate
    (*until December 31, 2023*)
CLAIRE BIFFL, Research Associate (*from January 1, 2024*)
RAYANE SILVA-CURRAN, Senior Program Assistant
KAVITA BERGER, Board Director, Board on Life Sciences
JULIE PAVLIN, Senior Board Director, Board on Global Health
CLARE STROUD, Senior Board Director, Board on
    Health Sciences Policy

Consultant

ELLEN CARLIN, Parapet Science & Policy Consulting

Reviewers

This Consensus Study Report was reviewed in draft form by individuals chosen for their diverse perspectives and technical expertise. The purpose of this independent review is to provide candid and critical comments that will assist the National Academies of Sciences, Engineering, and Medicine in making each published report as sound as possible and to ensure that it meets the institutional standards for quality, objectivity, evidence, and responsiveness to the study charge. The review comments and draft manuscript remain confidential to protect the integrity of the deliberative process.

We thank the following individuals for their review of this report:

DAVID BLAZES, Bill & Melinda Gates Foundation
MIKE BRAY, Georgetown Medical School
WILLIAM GREG BUREL, Hamilton Grace, LLC
JOHN H. CONNOR, National Emerging Infectious Diseases
    Laboratories, Boston University Chobanian and Avedisian School
    of Medicine
R. ALTA CHARO, University of Wisconsin–Madison
RICHARD HATCHETT, Coalition for Epidemic Preparedness
    Innovations
BERNARD MOSS, National Institutes of Health
UMAIR A. SHAH, Washington State Department of Health
ERICA SHENOY, Massachusetts General Hospital
JILL TAYLOR, Association of Public Health Laboratories
CRYSTAL WATSON, Johns Hopkins Bloomberg School
    of Public Health

Although the reviewers listed above provided many constructive comments and suggestions, they were not asked to endorse the conclusions or recommendations of this report, nor did they see the final draft before its release. The review of this report was overseen by **ANN M. ARVIN,** Stanford University, and **LAWRENCE COREY,** Fred Hutchinson Cancer Center. They were responsible for making certain that an independent examination of this report was carried out in accordance with the standards of the National Academies and that all review comments were carefully considered. Responsibility for the final content rests entirely with the authoring committee and the National Academies.

Contents

Boxes, Figures, and Tables

BOXES

FIGURES

TABLES

Preface

Immediately after the eradication of smallpox, nations around the world mobilized to ensure that future generations would not continue to suffer from this ancient and devastating disease. World Health Assembly resolution 33.4 declared that smallpox had been eradicated and recommended policies on vaccination, case investigation, and the limited retention of variola collections in the event of a future re-emergence. However, rapid societal, political, ecological, and technological changes of the 21st century have shed new light on these historical resolutions and the need to reevaluate public health and health systems capacities against natural and intentional threats. As evidenced by recent public health emergencies of international concern, the U.S. public—and the global community at large—expects the United States and its international partners, including the World Health Organization, to rapidly identify an outbreak and equitably make available safe and effective medical countermeasures (MCMs), such as effective diagnostics, therapeutics, biologics, and vaccines. These expectations hold true regardless of the pathogen causing the disease.

The National Academies of Sciences, Engineering, and Medicine's Committee on the Current State of Research, Development, and Stockpiling of Smallpox Medical Countermeasures was tasked with providing strategic counsel to the federal government and international partners regarding the future of the smallpox MCMs portfolio (including research, development, and stockpiling) to ensure readiness and effective response in the event of a smallpox event.

As articulated in this report, the committee envisions a responsive and flexible system to establish research priorities for smallpox MCMs, together with judicious stockpiling and strategic plans for the rapid and equitable distribution of MCMs in the event of a smallpox or other orthopoxvirus outbreak, in the United States or globally. Concurrently, the committee emphasizes the optimal use of governmental resources to achieve effective smallpox preparedness, while recognizing the competing demands placed on the government to also be prepared for other significant threats.

This type of system will require U.S. and international partners to plan and respond in the face of multiple scientific, societal, political, and ecological uncertainties. These uncertainties—and lessons learned from COVID and mpox—argue for research and stockpiling decisions to be made in anticipation of the next potential threat, with a readiness to shift priorities rapidly in the face of emerging information.

It is vital to prioritize research into and the development of safer and more effective MCMs, to make judicious choices about stockpiling, and to have modern, well rehearsed, and adaptable strategic plans in place to respond nationally and globally in the event of a variola or other orthopoxvirus outbreak. These efforts will depend on rapid identification (diagnostics and surveillance), effective containment and response, equitable allocation, and global solidarity.

On behalf of the committee and the project staff, I extend my sincere thanks to the many individuals who shared their time and expertise to support the committee's work and inform its deliberations. The study was sponsored by the Administration for Strategic Preparedness and Response on behalf of the U.S. government, and we thank Margaret Sloane and Julia Limage for their guidance and support. The committee extends great thanks and appreciation to Christy Huston of the U.S. Centers for Disease Control and Prevention and Rosamund Lewis of the World Health Organization Smallpox Secretariat for their technical advice. Our appreciation goes to the reviewers for their invaluable feedback and to the monitor and coordinator who oversaw the report review.

The committee acknowledges the many staff within the National Academies who provided support in various ways to this project, including Lisa Brown, Shalini Singaravelu, Matthew Masiello, Margaret McCarthy, Claire Biffl, and Rayane Silva-Curran. The committee also extends their gratitude to Clare Stroud, senior board director of the Board on Health Sciences Policy. Ellen Carlin provided research and writing assistance, Anne Marie Houppert assisted in compiling literature, and the report review, production, and communications staff all provided valuable guidance to ensure the success of the final product.

Finally, I would like to deeply thank the committee of experts who volunteered their invaluable time to this task. The committee's contributions to this report are reflective of their career-long dedication and service to epidemic and pandemic preparedness and response.

Lawrence O. Gostin, *Chair*
Committee on the Current State of Research, Development,
and Stockpiling of Smallpox Medical Countermeasures

Acronyms and Abbreviations

ACIP	Advisory Committee on Immunization Practices
ACVVR	Advisory Committee on Variola Virus Research
AI	artificial intelligence
AIDS	acquired immunodeficiency syndrome
APSV	Aventis Pasteur smallpox vaccine
ARPA-H	Advanced Research Projects Agency for Health
ASPR	Administration for Strategic Preparedness and Response
BARDA	Biomedical Advanced Research and Development Authority
BioMADE	BioIndustrial Manufacturing and Design Ecosystem
BioMaP	National Biopharmaceutical Manufacturing Partnership
CBRN	chemical, biological, radiological, and nuclear
CDC	U.S. Centers for Disease Control and Prevention
CDV	cidofovir
CEPI	Coalition for Epidemic Preparedness
CIADM	Centers for Innovation in Advanced Development and Manufacturing
CLIA	Clinical Laboratory Improvement Amendments
CMS	Centers for Medicare & Medicaid Services
CMV	cytomegalovirus
COVID-19	coronavirus disease 2019; the disease caused by the virus SARS-CoV-2
CRISPR	clustered regularly interspaced short palindromic repeats

DNA	deoxyribonucleic acid
DoD	Department of Defense
EA IND	expanded access for an investigational new drug
EIND	emergency investigational new drug
ELISA	enzyme-linked immunosorbent assay
EM	electron microscopy
EU	European Union
EUA	Emergency Use Authorization
EV	enveloped virion
FDA	U.S. Food and Drug Administration
FD&C	Food, Drug, and Cosmetic Act
FY	fiscal year
GAO	Government Accountability Office
GMP	good manufacturing practice
HERA	Health Emergency Preparedness and Response Authority
HHS	Department of Health and Human Services
HIV	human immunodeficiency virus
IgG	immunoglobulin G
IgM	immunoglobulin M
IND	investigational new drug
IOM	Institute of Medicine
IR	inverted repeat
ITAP	Independent Test Assessment Program
IV	intravenous
KFF	Kaiser Family Foundation
LAMP	loop mediated isothermal amplification
LDT	laboratory developed tests
LLM	large language model
LRN	Laboratory Response Network
mAbs	monoclonal antibodies
MCM	medical countermeasure
MERS-CoV	Middle East respiratory syndrome coronavirus
MPXV	monkeypox
mRNA	messenger ribonucleic acid
MV	mature virion

MVA	modified vaccinia Ankara
MVA-BN	modified vaccinia Ankara-Bavarian Nordic
NIAID	National Institute of Allergy and Infectious Diseases
NIH	National Institutes of Health
NYCBOH	New York City Board of Health
OPXV	orthopoxvirus
OWS	Operation Warp Speed
PCR	polymerase chain reaction
PHEMCE	Public Health Emergency Medical Countermeasures Enterprise
POC	point-of-care
PON	point-of-need
PPE	personal protective equipment
qPCR	quantitative polymerase chain reaction
SAGE	Strategic Advisory Group of Experts on Immunization
SARS	severe acute respiratory syndrome
SARS-CoV-2	severe acute respiratory syndrome-related coronavirus
SCARDA	Strategic Center of Biomedical Advanced Vaccine Research and Development for Preparedness and Response
SNS	U.S. Strategic National Stockpile
STOMP	Study of Tecovirimat for Human Monkeypox Virus
SVES	Smallpox Vaccine Emergency Stockpile
TPP	target product profile
VARV	variola virus
VECTOR	State Research Center of Virology and Biotechnology
VIG	vaccinia immunoglobulin
VIGIV	vaccinia immune globulin intravenous
WHA	World Health Assembly
WHO	World Health Organization

Acknowledgments

This Consensus Study Report would not have been possible without the many experts who generously contributed their time and expertise to inform the development of this report. The committee thanks all the speakers (Appendix A) for their timely participation and expert contributions to the public workshops: Steve Adams, Paul Chaplin, Matthew Clark, Gavin Cloherty, John Connor, Nicole Dorsey, Manoj Gandhi, Noel Gerald, Matthew Hepburn, Dennis Hruby, Nathaniel Hupert, Christy Hutson, Stuart Isaacs, Cyrus Javan, Ewa King, Brett Leav, Seth Lederman, Rosamund Lewis, Julia Limage, Karen Martins, Cathryn Mayes, Bernard Moss, Marcus Plescia, Chris Sinclair, Margaret Sloane, Crystal Watson, Daniel Wolfe, and Kevin Yeskey. The committee is deeply appreciative of the following individuals who contributed their expertise on poxvirus research: Jia Liu, Grant McFadden, Stefan Rothenburg, and Yan Xiang.

The committee would also like to thank the sponsor of this study. Funds for the committee's work was provided by the Administration for Strategic Preparedness and Response (ASPR). The committee also extends their gratitude to the group of interagency federal experts for informing the committee's charge.

Many others within the National Academies supported this project. The committee thanks the staff of the Health and Medicine Division (HMD) Executive Office, Office of Communications, Office of Governmental Affairs, and Research Center. The committee is grateful to Ellen Carlin for her invaluable contributions to conducting research, report writing, and editing. Finally, Robert Pool is to be credited for his editorial assistance in preparing this report.

We are deeply grateful to all those who collaborated on this project for working so diligently under a very short timeline.

Summary[1]

Smallpox—caused by variola virus, a member of the orthopoxvirus genus in the Poxviridae family—is an ancient disease that devastated humanity for millennia. In 1980 the World Health Assembly declared smallpox eradicated, and no naturally occurring smallpox cases have occurred since that time. There are only two known World Health Organization (WHO) sanctioned collections where variola virus samples are stored and used for research: the U.S. Centers for Disease Control and Prevention (CDC) in Atlanta, Georgia, and the State Research Center of Virology and Biotechnology (VECTOR) at Koltsovo in the Novosibirsk region of the Russian Federation. Yet, with advancements in genome amplification, sequencing, editing, and synthesis, it is now possible to recreate live smallpox virus from published genomes—raising the risks of both accidental and intentional releases. In other words, the destruction of known variola virus collections would no longer eliminate the threat of smallpox reemergence as a public health threat.

It therefore remains important to maintain robust public health and health system capacities and readiness to rapidly identify—and effectively respond to—a potential smallpox outbreak. Real-world experiences with outbreaks have revealed major challenges in medical countermeasure (MCM) development, manufacturing, distribution, and uptake, while also providing useful lessons and data points. Some smallpox MCMs have recently been deployed for mpox, including a third-generation smallpox vaccine and recently approved smallpox therapeutics. The coronavirus disease 2019 (COVID-19) pandemic ushered in advancements in MCM

---

[1] This Summary does not include references. Citations for the discussion presented in the Summary appear in the subsequent report chapters.

development and applicable technology that have potential applications for smallpox MCM development and utility.

The COVID-19 pandemic and mpox multi-country outbreak, both declared Public Health Emergencies of International Concern (PHEIC) by WHO, underscore the need for further domestic global coordination for preparedness and response against novel pathogens including orthopoxvirus events. At the request of the Administration for Strategic Preparedness and Response, on behalf of the U.S. government, the National Academies of Sciences, Engineering, and Medicine (the National Academies) was asked to convene an *ad hoc* committee to examine lessons learned from the COVID-19 pandemic and mpox outbreaks to inform an evaluation of the current state of research, development, and stockpiling of smallpox MCMs. The full charge to the committee is presented in Chapter 1. This report presents findings and conclusions that build on the Institute of Medicine's previous reports *Assessment of Future Scientific Needs for Live Variola Virus* (1999) and *Live Variola Virus: Considerations for Continuing Research* (2009) and serves to inform the position of the U.S. government for the upcoming 77th World Health Assembly in May 2024. This report does not contain recommendations.

STUDY APPROACH

The committee formulated seven overarching conclusions across two key aspects of smallpox readiness and response: (1) medical countermeasures readiness and (2) systems readiness. A set of more technical, chapter-specific conclusions based on the evidence are also presented in each chapter.

Discussions and conclusions on MCM readiness refer to having the "right" MCM or suite of MCMs available. Although the discussions on MCM readiness were primarily focused on those relevant for the U.S. population in a smallpox event, the committee emphasized the interdependence of the U.S. and international community in efforts to effectively contain any smallpox outbreak (Chapter 1). Understanding and reaching consensus on the right MCMs involved deliberations on the efficacy, effectiveness, and utility of the suite of different smallpox MCMs at various stages of development and stockpiling (Chapter 2). Additionally, the committee considered the future research and development that would be needed to improve existing smallpox MCMs, including research with live variola virus (Chapter 4).

Systems readiness discussions and conclusions refer to smallpox MCMs being available at the "right time" and for the "right people." The committee emphasizes the importance of not making the mistake of planning based on older response paradigms and challenges without taking into consideration new circumstances and possibilities and in Chapter 4 discusses future states of readiness for the MCM enterprise, including stockpiling considerations and international sharing of burden and benefit. To reach these future states, uncertainty and information about the evolving biothreat landscape, evolving technological landscape, societal factors, and operational considerations need to be accounted for in readiness and stockpiling approaches to ensure flexibility and adaptability (Chapter 3).

Challenges faced by the nation's MCM enterprise in efforts to rapidly scale and deploy MCMs during recent COVID-19 and mpox public health emergencies highlight urgent priorities that must be addressed to "future-proof" the nation's readiness and response postures against smallpox and other orthopoxviruses that may pose a biothreat.

OVERARCHING CONCLUSIONS ON MEDICAL COUNTERMEASURES READINESS

State of Smallpox MCM Readiness

A variety of MCMs have been developed to detect (diagnostics), prevent (vaccines), and treat (biological agents and antivirals) smallpox disease and transmission. Table S-1 lists the vaccines and therapeutics that are currently held in the U.S. Strategic National Stockpile (SNS). The SNS currently has sufficient live, replicating vaccine for the general population, a small amount of non-replicating vaccine for use in populations contraindicated for live replicating vaccine, and two smallpox antivirals with different mechanisms of action. While significant progress has been made to enhance the nation's readiness posture against smallpox since the disease was officially declared eradicated, challenges persist.

Gaps in the nation's readiness and response posture against unfamiliar pathogens were exposed during the COVID-19 pandemic and the 2022 mpox multi-country outbreak. One fundamental lesson learned from the COVID-19 and mpox emergencies is that research and development for new smallpox MCMs must not only consider the characteristics of the "product" but also must consider the ability to deploy at scale and ensure its equitable access.

The mpox outbreak, in particular, tested the MCMs that had been developed and stockpiled for smallpox against a related, but less lethal, orthopoxvirus. Regarding diagnosis, detection, and surveillance, challenges in scaling laboratory testing during COVID-19 and mpox limited the initial understanding of the scope and severity of these new and emerging threats, respectively. In the event of a smallpox outbreak, identification of cases would rely on clinical recognition, the availability of diagnostic assays at CDC Laboratory Response Network (LRN) laboratories, and potential to scale testing to points-of-care (POCs) or points-of-need (PONs), per the

TABLE S-1 Summary of Smallpox Vaccines and Therapeutics in the U.S. Strategic National Stockpile

Product Name	Characteristics and Details	Approved Usage or Indications
APSV (Wetvax)	1st generation Live, replicating vaccinia virus, NYCBOH-derived strain.	• Emergency Use Authorization (EUA)/investigational new drug (IND) for smallpox. • 1 dose regimen. • Multiple contraindications, especially for those who have immunocompromising, skin, or heart conditions. Contraindicated for those with serious allergy to a vaccine component.
ACAM2000	2nd generation Live, replicating vaccinia virus, NYCBOH-derived strain.	• FDA licensed for prevention of smallpox in all age groups for persons determined to be at high risk for smallpox infection. • 1 dose regimen. • Multiple contraindications, especially for those who have immunocompromising, skin, or heart conditions. Contraindicated for those with serious allergy to a vaccine component.
MVA-BN (Imvamune, Imvanex, JYNNEOS)	3rd generation Live, non-replicating vaccinia virus, MVA strain.	• FDA licensed for smallpox and mpox in adults 18 and older. • 2 dose regimen, 4 weeks apart. • Relatively few contraindications. Safely administered to individuals with immunocompromising, skin, or heart conditions. Contraindicated for those with serious allergy to a vaccine component.

Tecovirimat (ST-246/TPOXX)	Orthopoxvirus-specific inhibition of viral spread from cell to cell by targeting p37, a major envelope protein required for envelopment and excretion of extracellular forms of the virus.	• Treatment of smallpox (FDA approved).
		• Treatment of mpox under Investigational New Drug (IND), Expanded Access IND, Emergency IND (not FDA approved)
		  - STOMP/A5418 (Study of Tecovirimat for Human Mpox Virus)[a]
		  - STOMP sub-study of open label tecovirimat[b]
		  - Other Use: STOMP sub-study: Tecovirimat for Orthopox Virus Exposure[c]
		• No serious adverse events reported.

TABLE S-1 Continued

Product Name	Characteristics and Details	Approved Usage or Indications

Brincidofovir (CMX001/Tembexa)	Pro-drug of cidofovir; following phosphorylation of the prodrug to the active form cidofovir diphosphate, the drug targets the orthopoxvirus DNA polymerase, causing disruption of replication of the virus.	• Treatment of human smallpox infections only (FDA approved)
		 • Other uses[d] (EIND or EA IND):
		   - Study to Assess Brincidofovir Treatment of Serious Diseases or Conditions Caused by Double-Stranded DNA viruses[e] (phase 3 completed December 2022)
		   - Adenovirus in immuno-compromised persons: under clinical trial
		 • Potential for liver problems and increased risk for mortality with longer use. Potential for embryo-fetal toxicity, carcinogenicity, and male infertility based on animal studies.

Vaccinia Immune Globulin Intravenous Human (VIGIV) (CNJ-016)	Passive immunity for individuals with complications to vaccinia virus following vaccination; exact mechanism of action is not known.	• Treatment of complications due to vaccinia vaccination (FDA approved) • Other uses (EA IND): Potential use of stockpiled VIGIV for treatment of orthopoxviruses in an outbreak. • Contraindicated for individuals with history of anaphylaxis and cautioned for patients with renal insufficiency.

NOTES: Cidofovir (Vistide), another antiviral not currently stockpiled, targets orthopoxvirus DNA polymerase, causing disruption of replication of the virus. The licensed indication is for cytomegalovirus (CMV) retinitis and does not have licensed indication for OPXV/VARV therapy. However, it can be used "off label." Cidofovir was used in therapy of mpox in those with compromised immune systems/uncontrolled HIV during the 2022–2023 multi-country outbreak, as this treatment was commercially available. Potential side effects include renal toxicity.

CDC = U.S. Centers for Disease Control and Prevention; EA = expanded access; EIND = emergency investigational new drug; EUA = Emergency Use Authorization; FDA = U.S. Food and Drug Administration; IND = investigational new drug; OPXV = orthopoxvirus; VARV = variola virus.

[a] NIH/NIAID-sponsored: Phase 3 randomized, placebo-controlled, double-blind study to establish the efficacy of tecovirimat for the treatment of people with laboratory-confirmed or presumptive human monkeypox virus disease (HMPXV) [NCT05534984].

[b] Open label for pregnant or breastfeeding persons; those with severe immune suppression, significant skin conditions, or severe disease.

[c] For both mpox and smallpox for Department of Defense–affiliated personnel [NCT02080767].

[d] There are no registered clinical trials for brincidofovir at this time, could be used under EIND through CDC.

[e] Phase 3 trial completed 12/2022 with posted results [NCT01143181].

scale of the outbreak. The mpox experience also highlighted the increased demand for the third-generation, live, non-replicating vaccine, MVA-BN, given safety concerns for first- and second-generation smallpox vaccines that have been stockpiled at a higher quantity in the SNS. Furthermore, the mpox outbreak highlighted gaps in the smallpox therapeutic options, specifically on the reliance on challenge studies in animals and animal model data for understanding potential efficacy in humans and predicting antiviral resistance, and on a lack of diverse therapeutic options with distinct mechanisms of action.

For these reasons, the committee drew the following overarching conclusion:

1. The COVID-19 pandemic revealed weaknesses in the ability for the nation's public health and health care systems to rapidly and flexibly adapt the emergency response to an unfamiliar pathogen; whereas the 2022 mpox outbreak tested existing MCMs developed primarily for smallpox to contain a less lethal orthopoxvirus. The lessons learned from both emergencies call for strengthening the nation's laboratory response systems and further development of point-of-care diagnostics and genomics surveillance capabilities. Additionally, safer, single-dose vaccines and a diverse set of therapeutic options against smallpox would improve the U.S. readiness and response posture for immediate containment and long-term protection in a smallpox emergency.

Specific conclusions in Chapter 2 on diagnostics and surveillance (2-1), vaccines (2-2), and therapeutics (2-3) are below:

(2-1) Tests that can more accurately detect smallpox and other orthopoxviruses than those available today are needed; efforts should focus on (1) adapting multiplex nucleic acid assays for new platforms and field settings, (2) developing forward-deployed (POC/PON) assays to enhance equitable access to tests, including protein or antigen-based tests to rapidly test and isolate infected patients, (3) identifying FDA-approved serologic assays to assess individual and population levels of immunity against smallpox and history of related exposures, (4) validating nucleic acid testing using a variety of clinical samples, (5) developing different categories of laboratory tests for different biosafety levels, and (6) supporting a global network of laboratories to detect, diagnose, and conduct surveillance in humans and the environment.

(2-2) Smallpox vaccines that have improved safety across different population subgroups and are available as a single dose would support faster and more effective response to contain smallpox and other orthopoxvirus outbreaks. The development of novel smallpox vaccines using multi-vaccine platforms (i.e., use common vaccine vectors, manufacturing ingredients, and processes) would

improve the capacity for rapid vaccine production in response to a smallpox event and reduce the need for stockpiling in the SNS at current levels.

(2-3) To treat smallpox, the following would be advantageous to develop in order to supplement the therapeutic options currently approved and stockpiled in the SNS (1) new, safer antivirals with different and diverse targets, mechanisms of action, and routes of administration that minimize damage to host cells and have a high barrier to the development of resistance; (2) combination antiviral treatments and treatments based on novel technologies and platforms (e.g., genome editing, non-conventional targets, etc.); (3) vaccinia immune globulin intravenous (VIGIV) repurposed as part of combination therapy; (4) diverse options for non-vaccine biologics including monoclonal antibodies and antibody cocktails.

Evolving Biothreat and Technology Landscape

As the understanding of orthopoxviruses and biotechnologies advances, there is an opportunity to address the known gaps and deficiencies of MCMs against smallpox and other orthopoxviruses. Additionally, the range of risks and biothreats caused by orthopoxviruses and synthetic biology is broad, and the changing threat landscape is further evidenced by the increasing frequency and scope of orthopoxvirus outbreaks in recent years, including the first case of Alaskapox infection resulting in hospitalization and death and the recent increase of clade I mpox in the Democratic Republic of Congo (and with new cases in geographic areas that had not previously reported mpox).

For these reasons, the committee drew the following overarching conclusion:

2. **In addition to smallpox readiness, research should continue to be used to enhance readiness and response for other orthopoxviruses, this includes supporting the validation, approval and licensure, and commercialization of existing and next-generation MCMs for use in the management of non-variola orthopoxviruses as an efficient way to expand readiness more broadly by enabling vendor-managed inventory approaches to stockpiling.**

Conclusions in Chapter 2 (2-4) and Chapter 3 (3-1) on benefits to investing in orthopoxvirus research more broadly include:

(3-1) The increasing recognition of orthopoxvirus illnesses in humans merits ongoing research and development of MCMs to detect, prevent, treat, and respond to these diseases. This is of particular importance for mpox that is an ongoing global outbreak and is expected to be a long-term threat. Other emerging orthopoxviruses (e.g., Alaskapox, cowpox, and vaccinia-like viruses) also need

to be closely monitored as the population immunity against orthopoxviruses continues to wane.

(2-4) Most mpox therapeutics were developed because of investments in smallpox therapeutics, resulting in products found to have activity against mpox. Direct investment in developing therapeutics targeting circulating orthopoxviruses could similarly benefit smallpox therapeutic preparedness and could likely have more immediate utility and potentially achieve commercial viability.

As biotechnologies continue to evolve at a remarkable pace—a pace increasingly accelerated by major advances in artificial intelligence—it is incumbent on decision makers to consider what impacts and opportunities may arise in response to different MCM strategies. The malicious exploitation of such technologies to create novel bioterror agents could render an established MCM ineffective. Beneficial uses, if strategically developed and promulgated, could significantly mitigate infectious diseases as threats to personal, public, political, and environmental health. For these reasons, the committee drew the following overarching conclusion:

3. **A comprehensive and ongoing risk–benefit analysis is needed for smallpox MCMs research using emerging technologies as well as ongoing careful oversight to mitigate the risks of this research and ensure the risk–benefit balance is maintained.**

Conclusions in Chapter 3 on the implications of scientific and technological advancements on available smallpox MCMs (3-4, 3-5) include:

(3-4) The potential exists to synthesize the complete or partial variola virus genome and to manufacture infectious viral particles based on published genomes. Targeted modifications to the genome are also possible, which could alter functional components of the virus that could affect transmissibility or virulence. This capacity means that even the guaranteed complete eradication of all existing smallpox collections today would not guarantee against its reemergence as a threat. It also introduces greater challenges in readiness planning by introducing the possibility of atypical epidemiological or clinical presentations of the disease.

(3-5) Advances in emerging biotechnologies could also allow for the rapid development and deployment of MCMs. A global, real-time, distributed, manufacturing network could enable safe and equitable production of smallpox diagnostics, vaccines, and therapeutics when and where needed to rapidly bring an outbreak anywhere in the world under control. A strategic research and development program promoting the development of general capability in this regard has the potential to unlock such a future.

Smallpox Research Agenda

Orthopoxviruses can cause a spectrum of diseases, ranging from the very mild to the highly deadly, and understanding these distinctions requires understanding individual viruses. While there are advantages to conducting research with non-variola orthopoxviruses, these species cannot fully replace the knowledge gained by working with live variola virus. Research with live variola and non-variola orthopoxviruses informs the development of more precise smallpox diagnostics, supports the development of live virus vaccines and, ultimately, novel subunit vaccines or other innovations, and advances the development of therapeutics through improved understanding of viral functions and structures. In 1999 the Institute of Medicine (IOM) concluded:

> The most compelling need for long-term retention of live variola virus would be for the development of antiviral agents or novel vaccines to protect against a re-emergence of smallpox due to accidental or intentional release of variola virus.

IOM's 1999 finding that live virus is needed for certain aspects of research remains true today. For these reasons, the committee drew the following overarching conclusion:

4. **For the foreseeable future, some research with live variola virus remains essential to achieving public health research goals against an ever-evolving biothreat landscape and the potential for orthopoxviruses to emerge naturally or deliberately.**

In Chapter 4, Table 4-2 shows smallpox MCM readiness as a function of research with live variola and non-variola orthopoxviruses. It maps the potential for using these viruses or their components against specific knowledge gaps and MCM goals that could support improved public health benefit.

Conclusions in Chapter 3 (3-2, 3-3) and in Chapter 4 (4-1, 4-2) on a smallpox research agenda, including the utility of live variola virus research and clinical trial readiness (4-3), include:

> *(3-2) Variola virus-specific research is extremely restricted and is only undertaken when it is necessary and essential for public health. It is not possible to fill knowledge gaps without the study of other orthopoxviruses.*

> *(3-3) Gaps exist in the fundamental understanding of variola virus and non-variola orthopoxvirus biology, pathogenesis, immunity and host-interactions, evolution, transmission, and ecology. Basic poxvirus research is beneficial to smallpox MCM development and contributes to readiness against other known and potential novel orthopoxviruses affecting humans. General advances in*

developing orthopoxviruses as vaccine vectors, gene delivery, and oncolytic virotherapy can have multiple benefits, including enhancing smallpox MCMs.

(4-1) Research with live variola virus is essential for developing animal models to be used for MCM efficacy testing as a human surrogate, full verification of the potential efficacy of MCMs, and the development of certain targets for more effective therapeutic options, and it may be essential if advanced organoid or other sophisticated systems will be used to study these biologic interventions.

(4-2) Discovery research and pathogenesis research with live variola virus has merit as biomedical research without an immediate obvious connection to smallpox readiness and response.

(4-3) It is important to plan for clinical trials (e.g., of vaccine comparative effectiveness in conjunction with therapeutics and diagnostic testing) that will take place under real-world conditions during a smallpox outbreak to ensure that the following are in place: adaptive and streamlined trial designs, efforts toward diverse and equitable patient participation, and regulatory protocols that have been preapproved.

OVERALL CONCLUSIONS ON SYSTEMS READINESS

Operational Considerations for MCM Readiness and Stockpile Planning

Federal smallpox planning in the post-eradication era has been characterized by strategies to reduce the population risk that an outbreak would pose, primarily through containment using MCMs. The effectiveness of smallpox MCMs (whether diagnostics, vaccines, or therapeutics) as agents of risk reduction rests on numerous factors, from a working knowledge of smallpox biology, pathogenesis, and epidemiology to the risks and benefits of emerging science and technology, to myriad operational planning decisions. Chapter 3 briefly discusses operational planning issues related to manufacturing capacity, administration and uptake, frontline readiness and biosafety, and regulatory readiness. For these reasons, the committee drew the following overarching conclusion:

5. Readiness and response efforts involving MCMs are complex due to many factors. MCM development, stockpiling, and distribution planning must be flexible, adaptable, and robust against multiple potential smallpox event scenarios. Planning strategies should account for the complexities of each scenario and aim to support several health and well-being outcomes (e.g., health, justice, equity, and national/international demand).

The conclusions in Chapter 3 on operational considerations that influence readiness and response posture (3-6, 3-7, 3-8, 3-9, 3-10, 3-11, 3-12) are:

(3-6) The small number of manufacturers of smallpox MCMs is a readiness and response vulnerability—and it is clear there is insufficient capacity to scale MCM production in the event of a large-scale smallpox outbreak especially one of international scope.

(3-7) Given the lack of commercially available orthopoxvirus diagnostics, vaccines, and therapeutics, planning for logistics and supply chain management considerations is critical. Efforts could give consideration to developing plans to increase the number of smallpox vaccine and therapeutics manufacturers as well as optimizing current manufacturing capacities should they be needed in the shorter term.

(3-8) Communicating the risk and benefits of smallpox vaccination versus infection will be critically important. But experience with COVID-19 and mpox demonstrated that effective risk communication has been a challenge, especially considering vaccine hesitancy and the politicization of vaccination, and misinformation and disinformation. These same challenges could occur in a smallpox outbreak.

(3-9) Implementation research investigating the operational and social aspects of deploying and uptake of smallpox MCMs is needed to assess operational parameters that could affect readiness and response.

(3-10) Those on the front line—health care providers, public health practitioners and laboratorians, and first responders—need to have the capabilities and capacities to effectively and equitably diagnosis, prevent, and treat in the event of a smallpox outbreak. Clinical and public health guidance should be updated to reflect new data and new MCMs and should take into consideration the range of response strategies beyond post-exposure programs (i.e., ring vaccination).

(3-11) Regulatory readiness and responsiveness, applicable to all types of MCMs, will be critical in the event of a smallpox outbreak. This is especially relevant considering the additional laboratory biosafety concerns for smallpox compared with other orthopoxviruses.

(3-12) New regulatory models that can quickly evaluate MCMs that use novel platforms and newer methodologies need to be developed and implemented. This could be achieved through the sharing of necessary product characteristics, detailed submission requirements, and setting accepted benchmarks and immune assays (in the case of vaccines) ahead of time, as well as planning for surge staffing to ensure timely review and real-time engagement for inquiries.

The SNS and the Smallpox MCM Portfolio

A smallpox outbreak of any size (even a single case) will be initially perceived as an event of national and possible international (pandemic) potential, and the SNS will need to be forward leaning in its response until the source and scope of the outbreak are clear. Historically, the SNS has prioritized and devoted most of its resources to just two threats—smallpox and anthrax—and these threats remain substantive drivers of the SNS budget. As a result, the smallpox MCM portfolio is a relatively mature MCM portfolio that includes both prevention and treatment MCMs, and this is an advantage.

However, the 2022 mpox outbreak may hold specific relevance to SNS considerations. The successes of the mpox response were tempered by major challenges, especially the short supply of immediately available third generation licensed smallpox/mpox vaccine doses, as well as by concerns over needed changes in dosing and route of administration strategies not included in the vaccine's label for use during the outbreak response, inequitable access to vaccines and laboratory testing for patients, and overall federal, state, and local coordination.

To aid SNS administrators in their review of the future of the SNS smallpox MCM portfolio, the committee poses the considerations offered in Box S-1 (adapted from Box 4-2 in Chapter 4). To inform future priorities for the smallpox MCM portfolio, target product profiles (TPPs) for smallpox medical countermeasures could be developed (or in the case of smallpox vaccine, refined). This would include defining the product, including both the indication (i.e., disease/condition to be treated) and what an appropriate product would be to use in a public health emergency, prospectively establishing the metrics that define success for a product, and then building an experimental plan that assesses whether a product has critical attributes. Currently, the Biomedical Advanced Research and Development Agency (BARDA) has a TPP for smallpox vaccine, which could be refined and updated, and TPPs could be created for smallpox therapeutics and diagnostics. WHO also developed two diagnostic TPPs during the global mpox response and recommended that TPPs be developed for smallpox diagnostics.

While the existing stockpiling strategy has dramatically increased the baseline national readiness level for smallpox from an MCM perspective, the SNS is now more than two decades old and has several responses under its belt. The stockpile may be at an inflection point. As part of the SNS annual review process, transition plans could be established for mature MCM portfolios, such as smallpox. For these reasons, the committee drew the following overarching conclusion:

BOX S-1
Considerations for Smallpox MCMs in the SNS

High-Level Assessment

- *Articulating different goals and milestones depending on MCM portfolio maturity.* The smallpox MCM portfolio is a mature portfolio, and the goals of a mature portfolio should differ from a relatively new MCM portfolio.
- *Examining the potential uses of and implications for currently stockpiled MCMs for other orthopoxvirus outbreaks.* Consider the threat of other orthopoxviruses that stockpiled smallpox MCMs could be used for, and furthermore, if mpox becomes a more serious global health problem, consider the risk of further depletion of stockpiled smallpox MCMs.
- *Diversifying stockpiled smallpox MCMs.* The development and stockpiling of multiple MCMs may mitigate the risk of supply shortages and address potential efficacy, safety, pricing, administration, and uptake concerns, but it may also amplify sustainability concerns absent a commercial market for the products.
- *Developing a framework to guide decision making if new smallpox MCMs are developed.* For example, there is the possibility that assets for non-variola orthopoxviruses could appear on the market through private investment or the investment of other governments. The SNS will need a basis for considering whether and how these could support progress toward smallpox preparedness.
- *Optimizing maintenance and sustainment of current smallpox MCM stockpile.* As the SNS has shifted toward primarily sustaining the smallpox MCM stockpile, consider efforts and technology to reduce the cost of sustainment. For example, ongoing trials on freeze-dried formulation of MVA-BN could also present improved storage options for this vaccine compared with liquid formulation.
- *Reevaluating assumptions.* Stockpiling assumptions may need to consider the possibility of an increase or reduction in effective doses after potency testing against the disease-causing strain in an actual smallpox event. Similarly, ring vaccination or other vaccination strategies, vaccine hesitancy, and/or the existence of effective therapeutics might alter assumptions of a vaccine stockpile.
- *Planning for loss of manufacturing capacity.* Because the SNS relies on just a few manufacturers for smallpox MCMs, it is important to assess how a loss of manufacturing capacity from any given company could affect readiness and response and could inform strategies to ensure stability of the manufacturing base.

Operationalization: Rapid Deployment

- *Reviewing the deployment-ready stockpile formulation.* To ensure smallpox MCMs are ready to be deployed as quickly as possible.
- *Updating response plans and training and exercise tools to reflect current and potential new smallpox MCMs.* Consider issues such as multiple outbreak scenarios, triggers, and the scope of the required response (scalable plans and surge capacity). For example, plans may need to include how existing stockpiled vaccines would be used in the classic ring vaccination strategy or other vaccination strategies, and the number of doses needed, based on transmission of three to six new cases (reproductive number) from each case. Similarly, plans for the deployment of treatments based on exercised scenarios could further assist in defining short-term and longer-term needs during the emergency.

continued

BOX S-1 Continued

- *Planning for implementation, coordination, and communication considerations up front.* This may include research and development on topics such as logistics, equitable access and distribution of smallpox MCMs (allocation frameworks, transparent decision-making processes), information sharing, risk communication, and education and training for frontline responders.

MCM-Specific Stockpiling Considerations
- *Understanding the specific indications and requirements of each MCM* (e.g., supply sources/challenges; delivery needs; handling and storage requirements; shelf life and shelf-life extension, vendor-managed inventory, and optimal timing of administration for greatest efficacy; and adverse effects).

NOTE: This box was adapted from Box 4-2 in Chapter 4.

---

6. The smallpox MCM portfolio is a mature portfolio, and the goals of a mature portfolio should differ from a relatively new MCM portfolio. The scientific and technological opportunity for innovative and improved smallpox MCMs supports a transitional phase for the smallpox MCM portfolio, in which investments made to date are sustained to ensure a ready stockpile—while leveraging collaborations and partnerships with other nations and organizations to build a diversified smallpox MCM stockpile and an agile, on-demand, distributed MCM response network of the future.

Conclusions in Chapter 4 on strategies for smallpox MCM portfolio planning (4-4, 4-5, 4-6) include:

(4-4) The nation relies on the SNS to deploy MCMs in response to a smallpox event because, currently, most of the necessary MCMs are not commercially available. Moving forward, leveraging collaborations and partnerships with other nations and organizations to develop next-generation smallpox and orthopoxvirus MCMs and expanding the use of the current ones could create a shared burden and enable a pathway toward international sharing of benefits.

(4-5) To facilitate a successful response in the event of a smallpox outbreak, the suite of smallpox MCMs (diagnostics, vaccines, and therapeutics) will be deployed and must work in concert with one another. However, the smallpox MCM suite has not been tested or exercised in this way: These MCMs were not used during the smallpox eradication campaign, some have not been deployed simultaneously before, and some are based on older technology and use outdated assumptions, including changes in population (e.g., demographic, physiological, and behavioral/risk perception).

(4-6) Threat assessments and specific response scenarios, based on different potential smallpox or orthopoxvirus events, are needed to assess and determine the necessary quantities and types of MCMs needed for various effective and equitable response strategies (e.g., early detection, immediate versus long-term response, isolation of patients, quarantine of contacts, use of therapeutics for prophylaxis and treatment including pre-exposure prophylaxis with therapeutics for first responders and health care providers, ring vaccination, or mass vaccination).

Global Cooperation

The COVID-19 pandemic and the mpox multi-country outbreak demonstrated the speed with which biothreats occurring internationally can affect and overwhelm national medical and public health response systems. These events also highlighted the shortfalls of the global MCM enterprise in ensuring equitable access to MCMs in the United States and globally, along with enduring concerns about public acceptability of countermeasures, presented a challenge in containing disease transmission around the globe. For these reasons the committee drew the following overarching conclusion:

7. **In a smallpox event, the U.S. readiness and response posture will be significantly affected by the ability of other countries around the world to adequately detect smallpox and contain transmission. Given global interdependence and global supply chains, supporting MCM capacities and capabilities internationally (i.e., a global MCM platform) will improve security against biothreats in the United States.**

Specific conclusions in Chapter 1 on the implications of the U.S. smallpox MCM enterprise for potential global smallpox events (1-1, 1-2) are:

(1-1) The ability for many countries to contain a smallpox outbreak is currently dependent on the U.S. readiness and response posture to rapidly deploy MCMs upon request and in collaboration with WHO and global partners. Thus, U.S. stockpiling decisions must take international commitments and equity arrangements into account.

(1-2) The U.S. pledge of smallpox vaccines to the WHO Smallpox Vaccine Emergency Stockpile (SVES) represents a substantial proportion of what has been promised by WHO Member States. However, the number of doses in the SVES would likely be inadequate for a global response and would require additional MCMs to be produced to meet the demands of a response to deliver equitable access globally.

CONCLUDING REMARKS

A smallpox outbreak, regardless of whether it happens in the United States or in other countries, would pose a major public health and security threat and would create considerable public expectations of an effective and timely response. Findings from studies of past public health emergencies indicated a lack of adequate public health and health system readiness and response capabilities, the importance of global cooperation and collaboration, and the need to think beyond a "one-pathogen" approach.

The United States maintains a national MCM stockpile and plans to diagnose, prevent, and treat smallpox. Despite the research done over recent decades and the fact that there are more smallpox MCMs available now than there were in the pre-eradication period, the nation's readiness and response posture to a smallpox event could be strengthened. These MCM assets and the plans designed to make use of them must be continually updated and forward-looking to account for changes in science and technology, populations at risk, and geopolitical factors. The committee envisions that the priorities set forth in this report and summarized in Box S-2 contribute to society's ability to prepare for and respond to a potential smallpox event.

BOX S-2
Summary of Priorities for Improved Smallpox Readiness and Response

The following points collectively summarize at a high-level the priorities identified by the committee that are needed to improve the smallpox readiness and response posture.

Medical Countermeasures Readiness
- **Smallpox Research Agenda** – Research and development roadmap for live variola virus research and pathways to support the validation, approval and licensure, and commercialization of existing and next-generation MCMs for use in the management of non-variola orthopoxviruses.
- **Diagnostics and Surveillance** – Expanded diagnostics and surveillance supported by (1) multiplex nucleic acid assays for new platforms, field settings, and for use with clinical samples prior to onset of rash illness; (2) forward-deployed point-of-care assays including protein- or antigen-based tests to rapidly test and isolate infected patients; (3) FDA-approved serologic assays to assess individual and population levels of immunity against smallpox and history of exposures.
- **Vaccines** – Safe and efficacious single-dose smallpox vaccines that (1) have utility for immediate outbreak containment as well as long-term protection, and (2) can be quickly adapted and developed at scale if needed to protect against a novel strain.
- **Therapeutics** – Diverse, safer smallpox therapeutics options including (1) antivirals with different and diverse targets, mechanisms of action, and routes of administration; (2) combination antiviral treatments and treatments based on novel technologies and platforms (e.g., genome editing, non-conventional targets, etc.); (3) vaccinia immune globulin intravenous (VIGIV) repurposed as part of combination therapy; (4) diverse options for non-vaccine biologics including monoclonal antibodies and antibody cocktails.
- **Emerging Technologies** – Ongoing risk/benefit analysis conducted periodically for smallpox MCM research and development using emerging technologies.

Systems Readiness
- **Operational Considerations** – Periodic assessment of implementation and operational factors that might influence smallpox readiness and response, including manufacturing capacity, frontline readiness, risk communication, and regulatory readiness.
- **Strategic National Stockpile** – Transition plan for the smallpox MCM portfolio, in which investments made to date are sustained to ensure a ready stockpile—while working with other nations and organizations to build a diversified smallpox MCM stockpile and an agile, on-demand, distributed response MCM network of the future. Budgetary stress on stockpile purchases and maintenance could be reduced through the commercialization of these smallpox MCMs for non-variola orthopoxviruses.
- **Global Cooperation** – U.S. investment and support in MCM research, development, and deployment capacities and capabilities internationally.

1

Introduction

"*The price of freedom from smallpox disease is eternal vigilance.*"
Oyewale Tomori, International
Congress of Virology, 1993

Smallpox has long been feared as a lethal and disfiguring disease (Henderson, 2009). The global smallpox eradication achievements at the end of the 20th century set in motion preparedness efforts designed to quickly contain any natural, accidental, or deliberate emergence. Since the eradication of naturally occurring smallpox more than four decades ago, remaining collections of variola virus and advancements in genome amplification, sequencing, editing, and synthesis have presented both a danger to and safeguard of a world free from smallpox. Lessons learned from recent public health emergencies shed new light on vulnerabilities in the nation's readiness to swiftly contain emerging infectious disease threats, which calls into question the historical assumptions that underpin the smallpox medical countermeasures (MCMs) portfolio. New evidence from the use of smallpox in response to the 2022 multi-country mpox outbreaks, including administration of third-generation vaccines and recently approved therapeutics, may provide further insight to the utility of these MCMs against smallpox should it re-emerge. Moreover, the coronavirus disease 2019 (COVID-19) pandemic ushered in advancements in MCM technology and developments that have potential applications for smallpox MCMs. Simultaneously, major challenges in MCM development, manufacturing, distribution, and uptake surfaced during the response to COVID-19 that will have implications for future smallpox readiness and response.

The World Health Organization (WHO) Advisory Committee on Variola Virus Research (ACVVR) recently noted that "preparedness for smallpox is currently inadequate, that equitable provision of countermeasures was not achieved during the global mpox outbreak, and that the global community must further invest in supporting access to resources arising from the variola virus research programme monitored by WHO" (WHO, 2024). Despite the importance of these recent lessons, the committee also emphasizes the importance of not "fighting the last war," or making the mistake of planning based on old challenges without taking into consideration new circumstances and possibilities.

RATIONALE AND STUDY CHARGE

Federal responsibility in the United States for maintaining a stockpile of MCMs to address smallpox and other threats lies with the Administration for Strategic Preparedness and Response (ASPR), an operating division of the Department of Health and Human Services (HHS). The U.S. Strategic National Stockpile, or SNS, contains smallpox vaccines, drugs, and related supplies and medical devices that the secretary of HHS can deploy to state, local, tribal, and territorial jurisdictions at their request in the event of a smallpox emergency (Kuiken and Gottron, 2023). HHS has also pledged a proportion of its smallpox vaccine for international use since 2004 (BioSpace, 2004).

Work with variola virus for research at the two WHO collaborating centers with official collections of variola, the U.S. Centers for Disease Control and Prevention (CDC) and State Research Center of Virology and Biotechnology (VECTOR) in Koltsovo, Russia, has been overseen by the ACVVR since a 1999 World Health Assembly (WHA) decision (WHA52.10) to authorize the temporary retention of remaining collections (WHO, 1999). Work with live variola virus and its genes is limited in scope and highly regulated by WHO. ACVVR oversees research using live variola virus and approves or rejects research proposals with live virus, discussed further in Chapter 3 (Box 3-1).

ASPR requested that the National Academies of Sciences, Engineering, and Medicine (National Academies) evaluate the current state of smallpox MCMs and implications for the SNS to inform the development of the U.S. government position and deliberations at the 77th World Health Assembly (see the statement of task in Box 1-1). Outcomes of this analysis can help ASPR reach an up-to-date understanding of smallpox MCM readiness and response in the context of these experiences, consider changes to its stockpiling strategy that can optimize a robust public health response, and develop research priorities that can help achieve that aim. This report builds on the Institute of Medicine's (IOM's) previous reports *Assessment*

BOX 1-1
Statement of Task

An ad hoc committee of the National Academies of Sciences, Engineering, and Medicine will conduct a study to examine lessons learned from the recent coronavirus disease 2019 (COVID-19) pandemic and mpox multi-country outbreak to inform an evaluation of the current state of research, development, and stockpiling of smallpox medical countermeasures (MCMs). The committee will:

1. Consider how the COVID-19 pandemic and the mpox multi-country outbreak can inform improvements to smallpox readiness and response, including the availability of smallpox MCMs and the ability to meet potential demand.
2. Examine the current state of MCMs for the diagnosis, prevention, and treatment of smallpox, including:
   a. How the mpox outbreak altered assumptions about the efficacy and utility of smallpox MCMs.
   b. The continued role of live variola virus for research and public health purposes.
   c. Implications for the composition of smallpox MCMs in the U.S. Strategic National Stockpile (SNS).
3. Explore the benefits and risks of scientific and technological advances on smallpox readiness and response and identify key priorities in research and development of smallpox MCMs.

Building on the Institute of Medicine's previous reports, *Assessment of Future Scientific Needs for Live Variola Virus* (1999) and *Live Variola Virus: Considerations for Continuing Research* (2009), and a review of existing literature, analyses, and other expert and public input, the committee will develop a report with its findings and conclusions on priorities for additional research or activities to improve the U.S. government readiness and response posture against smallpox, and on the composition of the SNS to ensure appropriate smallpox MCM response options.

---

of Future Scientific Needs for Live Variola Virus (1999) and *Live Variola Virus: Considerations for Continuing Research* (2009). The committee was asked to provide only conclusions, not recommendations, on priorities for additional research or activities to improve smallpox readiness and response posture.

To address its charge, the National Academies convened a committee of experts comprising 14 members with academic backgrounds and professional expertise in fields including molecular microbiology and immunology; virology; infectious disease and health care; public health preparedness and epidemiology; vaccine and drug research, development, and production; medical countermeasures; whole-genome sequencing and diagnostic technologies; biosecurity and biosafety; emerging technologies; biomedical and public health ethics; and risk assessment. Appendix B provides the biographies of the committee members.

ABOUT THIS REPORT

Study Approach

In developing this report and the conclusions presented herein, the committee deliberated from November 2023 through February 2024 and held five virtual meetings. The committee heard from subject-matter experts across the federal government, industry, academia, and professional associations on key lessons and opportunities for smallpox readiness and response during multiple open session days (all public meeting agendas can be found in Appendix A). The committee and National Academies staff also conducted a review of literature published since 2009 and were informed by reports and deliberations of the 154th session of the WHO Executive Board.

Study Scope

The committee was asked to examine the utility of smallpox MCMs and implications for smallpox readiness and response considering lessons learned from recent public health emergencies. Further clarification during open session meetings with the sponsor tasked the committee to specifically consider strategic approaches for stockpiling smallpox MCMs and an enumeration of the ways in which research using live variola virus could provide benefits in a smallpox emergency (Sloane, 2023).

This report does not address the special challenges with developing vaccines and therapeutics for special populations, such as pediatric populations, pregnant and lactating persons, or immunocompromised persons. There are clearly challenges associated with developing vaccines and therapeutics for special populations—which may not always mean something as simple as dose reduction or schedule modification. Development of such products suitable for these populations will require close consultation with regulators.

It is important to note that the committee was not asked to decide about the destruction or retention of live variola virus collections; such a determination involves information beyond the purview of the committee. The committee was also not asked to conduct detailed assessments of the threat and potential for a smallpox outbreak, the risks of live variola virus research, or the risks of dual-use research of concern. The committee supports the position that any research with live variola virus requires rigorous scientific evaluation before being conducted as well as necessary laboratory safeguards to protect researchers and the public and proper infrastructure and research capacity. Lastly, this report does not contain recommendations.

Report Audiences and Key Stakeholders

This report is intended for the immediate use, by request, of ASPR on behalf of the U.S. government. However, there are a variety of domestic and global stakeholders involved in the smallpox MCM enterprise (Figure 1-1), and the committee designed this report to help these stakeholders understand and use available information to inform their decision making. Smallpox readiness and stockpiling decisions must account for the threat

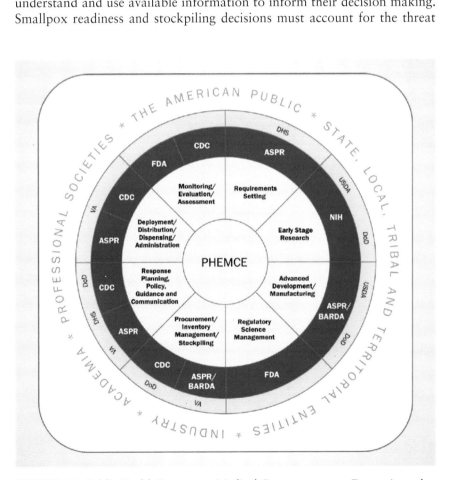

FIGURE 1-1 Public Health Emergency Medical Countermeasures Enterprise stakeholders and engagement.
SOURCES: NASEM (2021). Originally from Korch (2016).

of a smallpox outbreak; the ability to detect and confirm cases; the ability to develop and manufacture MCMs for large populations; approvals from regulatory agencies for new or updated MCMs; the availability, rapid deployment, and uptake of smallpox MCMs; and the public's understanding of the threat and their acceptance of the offered MCMs. Ultimately, effective uptake and utilization of MCMs depends on the willingness and health-seeking behaviors of the affected public and the interactions between them and the public health agencies and health care providers responsible for dispensing and administering MCMs. The audience for this report includes:

- Public Health Emergency Medical Countermeasures Enterprise (PHEMCE) and other federal partners like the Advanced Research Projects Agency for Health (ARPA-H)
- Federal policy makers, including members of Congress
- State, tribal, local, and territorial officials and policy makers
- Industry, including suppliers, manufacturers, and distributors
- Health systems and public health agencies
- Public health practitioners and laboratorians, first responders, and health care providers
- General public
- Researchers, especially those who participate in the research agenda on variola virus and other orthopoxviruses (CDC, National Institutes of Health [NIH], U.S. Food and Drug Administration [FDA], Department of Defense [DoD], academic centers, and international partners)
- Guidance-setting organizations and groups (e.g., CDC Advisory Committee on Immunization Practices [ACIP], WHO Strategic Advisory Group of Experts on Immunization [SAGE] for smallpox and mpox vaccines, etc.)
- International partners, including WHO and other countries
- Public, private, philanthropic, civil society organizations, and professional societies with a vested interest in the MCM enterprise

Report Organization

Chapter 1 discusses the high-level lessons learned from past public health emergencies, lessons in global cooperation, and potential emergence and response factors. Chapter 2 introduces the MCMs developed to detect, prevent, and protect against smallpox in the post-eradication era, within the context of potential smallpox containment strategies. Chapter 3 discusses factors that may influence stockpiling considerations as well as other readiness planning decisions, including the impacts of orthopoxvirus characteristics, emerging technologies, and operational considerations on the development, testing, and deployment of smallpox MCMs. Chapter 3 also clarifies differences in viral characteristics and impacts in humans for the *Poxviridae* family of viruses and the *Orthopoxvirus* genus that primarily affects humans. While this report focuses on orthopoxviruses, their potential to cause disease in humans, and MCMs developed against them, the committee recognizes the potential for spillover of other poxviruses to occur from animal reservoirs to humans. Chapter 4 presents ways forward to address gaps in research, understanding, and effectiveness of smallpox MCM options developed to date as well as considerations to inform stockpiling strategies.

BACKGROUND AND CONTEXT

Smallpox Research and Medical Countermeasures Post-Eradication

Following the success of the globally coordinated WHO smallpox eradication program, WHA declared smallpox eradicated in 1980 after the last natural case occurred in 1977 (Fenner et al., 1988). In the post-eradication era, resolution WHA33.4 (1980) recommended measures for Member States to implement if smallpox should reemerge (WHO, 1980). Subsequent WHA resolutions directed the consolidation of remaining variola virus collections to two official locations: CDC in Atlanta, Georgia, and the VECTOR Institute in Koltsovo, Russia, with ACVVR oversight of research using variola virus (WHO, 2007, 2016).

Following a 1986 recommendation of the WHO Ad Hoc Committee on Orthopoxvirus Infections to destroy the remaining viral specimens, the WHA set the date for the destruction of the live variola virus collections on June 30, 1999 (WHO, 1986, 1996). Implementation of that decision, however, has been deferred ever since in part based on a justification that the live viruses were needed to support further research and development of medical countermeasures to defend against natural, accidental, or intentional smallpox reemergence (IOM, 2009; WHO, 1999).

Global and U.S. Smallpox Medical Countermeasures Stockpiles

In 1980, WHA Resolution 33.4 recommended the establishment of a physical international reserve of smallpox vaccines, to be known as the Smallpox Vaccine Emergency Stockpile (SVES), comprising remaining vaccine doses from the Smallpox Eradication Program and additional WHO Member State donations (WHO, 1980, 2017). In 1999, the U.S. Congress directed CDC to establish a U.S. national pharmaceutical and vaccine stockpile for biological and chemical threats. The Department of Homeland Security determined smallpox, among other pathogens, to be "material threats" to national security following the September 11, 2001, terrorist attacks on the United States. Originally known as the National

Pharmaceutical Stockpile, a 2002 law changed its name to the SNS and further defined and expanded its mandate (Kuiken and Gottron, 2023). An interagency working group, PHEMCE, was established in the ensuing years to inform HHS decisions in determining which threats to stockpile against, including pandemic influenza, viral hemorrhagic fevers, antibiotic resistant bacteria, chemical threats, radiological and nuclear threats, ancillary supplies, and other targets and materiel (NASEM, 2021).

Early domestic smallpox preparedness efforts coincided with pledges from the United States and other countries to contribute doses of smallpox vaccine to a "virtual global stockpile of pledged vaccine from around the world," pursuant to the adoption of WHA55.16 in 2002 (CIDRAP, 2004). That resolution urged WHO Member States to share expertise, supplies, and resources in a global public health emergency (CIDRAP, 2004; WHO, 2002, 2017). The United States has maintained its commitment to the global smallpox vaccine stockpile, having affirmed its pledged vaccines for 20 million people in 2024 in advance of the 154th session of the WHO Executive Board (Lewis, 2023). The pledged vaccines are held in the SNS and are intended to be made available to WHO in the event of a smallpox emergency outside the United States (BioSpace, 2004). The donation would be a mix of all three vaccines held in the SNS in proportions that they are represented at the time.[1]

To obtain vaccine through the WHO SVES, a WHO Member State requests vaccine from WHO; WHO then decides on the type, quantity, and deployment of vaccines and arranges for importation, while the requesting country obtains authorization for use of the vaccine products and ancillary supplies locally. If a given vaccine lacks market authorization in either the donor or recipient country, the national regulatory authority of the requesting country must be prepared to conduct an emergency assessment (WHO, 2017). Discussions on the composition of the WHO SVES reopened in 2021 to consider the addition of antivirals and diagnostics in virtual stockpile agreements, however these negotiations were delayed by the 2022 mpox multi-country outbreak and only recently resumed (Lewis, 2023).

Conclusions on Global Stockpiling

Based on the above evidence and findings, the committee drew the following conclusions:

(1-1) The ability for many countries to contain a smallpox outbreak is currently dependent on the U.S. readiness and response posture to rapidly deploy MCMs upon request and in collaboration with WHO and

---

[1] Personal communication, Margaret Sloane, Administration for Strategic Preparedness and Response (ASPR), January 16, 2024.

global partners. Thus, U.S. stockpiling decisions must take international commitments and equity arrangements into account.

(1-2) The U.S. pledge of smallpox vaccines to the WHO Smallpox Vaccine Emergency Stockpile (SVES) represents a substantial proportion of what has been promised by WHO Member States. However, the number of doses in the SVES would likely be inadequate for a global response and would require additional MCMs to be produced to meet the demands of a response to deliver equitable access globally.

LESSONS LEARNED FROM RESPONDING TO COVID-19 AND MPOX

ASPR asked the committee to consider lessons learned from COVID-19 and mpox in its thinking about how national smallpox MCM assets could be optimized. The initial response failures to COVID-19 in the United States have been attributed to "the nation's pre-existing structural and systemic features, which magnified the pandemic's impact" as well as failures in government at many levels "to generate reliable information, communicate it in a timely and consistent manner, and translate it into sound policy" (Yamey et al., 2024).

Diagnostic Availability and Testing Delays

From the beginning of the COVID-19 pandemic, the United States quickly experienced a bottleneck in testing capacity as it attempted to respond. The U.S. delay in rolling out and scaling up laboratory-based testing was marked compared to the experiences of other countries. According to Our World in Data, a nonprofit that collated data from WHO and other sources, Argentina and Mexico reported starting testing individuals at single-digit levels in the second week of January 2020, followed by Taiwan and Thailand later that month. On February 5, Hong Kong reported 124 tests; South Korea followed by mid-February and quickly ramped up to hundreds of tests per day (Our World in Data, 2020). CDC was subject to extensive criticism for the delays in early testing. In its own after-action report, the agency identified contamination, poor design, and problems with quality control as proximal culprits, with inadequate planning, inadequate governance, and a failed incident management structure as fundamentally contributing factors (CDC, 2023). The advisory group that drafted the report issued a series of recommendations related to laboratory and testing leadership, oversight, and exercising.

Once laboratory tests were up and running, it became clear that a significant level of potential testing capacity was going unused. Many academic molecular biology laboratories pivoted their focus to become certified testing laboratories but found in the spring of 2020 that they were nowhere near reaching throughput capacity despite significant wait times for test results. Hospitals and clinics were sending their samples to laboratories with which they had preexisting contracts and compatible health record software (Maxmen, 2020).

FDA authorized the first rapid COVID-19 test for at-home self-testing on November 17, 2020, through an Emergency Use Authorization (EUA) (FDA, 2020a). A sudden increase in the need for diagnostic testing in the face of new highly transmissible variants, such as Omicron, challenged both public and private laboratories as well as testing manufacturers (O'Donnell and Abouleneim, 2021; Smyth et al., 2022), and highlighted the importance of maintaining a large surge capacity. Some experts have argued that earlier research and development investment in years prior to the pandemic could have strengthened the fundamental science and knowledge base that would have supported quicker rapid diagnostic availability (Bipartisan Commission on Biodefense, November 2020). In addition to the need for greater surge testing capacity, COVID-19 underscored the importance of maintaining a cadre of public health laboratory workforce and a dedicated supply chain for diagnostic test manufacturing, sample collection, and processing, (Behnam et al., 2020; Wolford et al., 2023).

Unlike the development of novel COVID-19 diagnostics, the development of mpox diagnostics had occurred decades prior to the 2022 U.S. outbreak as part of global recommendations for smallpox preparedness (Cahill, 2023). No point-of-care diagnostics were available, but the science to support laboratory diagnosis of mpox was robust. Many laboratory-based tests have been described in the literature, including real-time polymerase chain reaction (PCR) assays used for mpox (Li et al., 2006, 2010) and an enzyme-linked immunoassay used on subjects from Wisconsin (Karem et al., 2005), the epicenter of the 2003 U.S. outbreak, as just a few examples. Two CDC-developed and FDA-approved real-time PCR laboratory test kits were already in use at Laboratory Response Network (LRN) laboratories. This differential availability of testing speaks to the investments made in known pathogens, including a designated material threat, compared to a novel infectious pathogen and one from a viral family that had received minimal attention.

Despite the existence of FDA-approved test kits for mpox, testing during the 2022 multi-country outbreak was initially slow for the scope of the emergency. Frustration among doctors and patients over testing was common early on in the 2022 U.S. mpox outbreak. The *Journal of the American Medical Association* reported that despite availability of 8,000 tests weekly through upward of 67 public health labs, clinicians faced a cumbersome process in ordering tests (Suran, 2022). Testing was initially limited to LRN laboratories, and although commercial testing ramped up by late summer, some felt it was too slow and that the government was repeating the mistakes of COVID-19 (Lewis, 2022). One of the limiting factors for expansion of testing was the lack of diversity of testing assays and platforms at the beginning of the outbreak. Once again supply chain for materials presented a challenge, making LRN sites depedent on manual nucleic acid extraction kits from one manufacturer which could be used with the FDA 510(k) cleared assay (Wolford et al., 2023).

Once reagents and automation were added, availability was expanded to several commercial labs by June 2022. Testing capacity would reach 80,000 per week by July 2022 (CDC, 2022). On September 7, after an official declaration of a public health emergency, FDA issued EUA authorities to further expand in vitro diagnostic testing availability for monkeypox virus; the declaration was drafted broadly to include testing options that detect or diagnose infection with non-variola orthopoxvirus (FDA, 2023b). Moving forward, collaboration and communication between CDC and FDA would help the agencies expand the use of the CDC-approved orthopoxvirus laboratory test (Gerald, 2023).

Between September 2022 and March 2023, eight additional tests were authorized under EUA: three automated laboratory tests; two automated point-of-care tests; one lab-based test with high daily testing capacity; and two manual test kits that used different reagents and instrumentation (Gerald, 2023). FDA's goal with these approvals was to reduce reliance on single platforms. The Independent Test Assessment Program (ITAP), established as part of NIH's Rapid Acceleration of Diagnostics (RADx) Tech program to support the COVID-19 response, was pivotal in bringing some of these mpox tests to market (NIBIB, n.d.). ITAP's purpose was to accelerate regulatory review of accurate and reliable diagnostics, initially during the COVID-19 crisis and continuing to support mpox diagnostics (NIBIB, 2022). The first point-of-care test for mpox (Xpert Mpox by Cepheid) received EUA in February 2023 with the support of ITAP (FDA, 2023b).

Vaccine and Therapeutic Availability, Access, and Uptake

The successes of Operation Warp Speed (Chapter 3) in developing safe and effective vaccines in record time were tempered by major issues with accessibility and uptake domestically and globally. While the foundations of coronavirus research, on which COVID-19 vaccine was developed, was anchored largely in post-SARS investment by NIH, some experts have questioned whether we would have been as ready for a virus from another family (Branswell, 2022), and note an overall lack of revolutionary, intergovernmental effort on MCMs for emerging infectious diseases until the nation was in crisis (Bipartisan Commission on Biodefense, 2021). Additionally, while mRNA-based COVID-19 vaccines helped reduce serious illness and hospitalization, an unanticipated level of vaccine hesitancy and vaccine related mis- and dis-information hampered uptake and had not been planned for.

Clinical trial networks to test therapeutics against COVID-19 enabled rapid recruitment for intensive care unit patients, however some argued that the lack of an established framework outside of intensive care unit patients to support clinical trials was a significant challenge that led to small, underpowered studies with repurposed drugs (Robinson et al., 2022). This resulted in limited insight into pre- or post-hospital stages of COVID-19 through these trials. Moving forward, some argued that a government established and organized network of hospitals for large clinical trial implementation and rapid data sharing could have produced more answers and potentially more solutions for health care providers who faced a high burden of hospitalizations with very few therapeutic tools (Zimmer, 2021).

In May 2020, FDA issued an EUA for Veklury (Remdesivir), an existing antiviral repurposed for SARS-CoV-2; the agency granted full approval in October of that year under Fast Track and Priority Review designations and provided the company a Material Threat Medical Countermeasure Priority Review Voucher (FDA, 2020b). Ultimately, FDA provided full approval for three additional drugs for the treatment of COVID: Actemra (Tocilizumab) and Olumiant (baricitinib), both repurposed, and Paxlovid (nirmatrelvir and ritonavir), a novel combination of one new antiviral and one existing HIV protease inhibitor. Remdesivir, Tocilizumab, and baricitinib received indications for hospitalized patients, while Paxlovid as well as Remdesivir were indicated for mild to moderate COVID-19 cases at high risk for progression. Other drugs were available on an EUA basis.

A 2022 Kaiser Family Foundation analysis of Paxlovid and another oral therapy being used under an EUA, Lagevrio (molnupiravir), found disparities in access to at-home orally administered treatments in the United States, with impoverished counties and those that were majority Black, Hispanic, or American Indian or Alaska Native facing reduced access—the same populations that disproportionately suffered poor COVID-19 outcomes (Hill et al., 2022; Leggat-Barr et al., 2021; Magesh et al., 2021).

The potential role of effective therapeutics was salient in a pandemic characterized by a concerning level of vaccine hesitancy. The relationship between vaccine and antiviral hesitancy appears complex. One analysis found that Paxlovid use (but not Lagevrio) was higher in states with higher vaccination rates (Murphy et al., 2022). On the other hand, more anecdotal reports indicate a greater acceptance of therapeutics among some with anti-vaccine tendencies (Craven, 2021; Facher, 2022). Understanding the dynamic interplay between vaccine and therapeutic acceptance will be important for modeling acceptance scenarios for smallpox MCMs.

In marked contrast to the start of the COVID-19 pandemic, the U.S. government had stockpiled MCMs that would be effective to respond to the 2022 mpox multi-country outbreak through the SNS smallpox MCMs portoflio. Specifically, the SNS had stockpiles of modified vaccinia Ankara vaccine developed by Bavarian Nordic (MVA-BN), an attenuated live, non-replicating vaccine indicated for smallpox and mpox (ASPR, n.d.;

FDA, 2023a). MVA-BN had received full FDA approval for the prevention of smallpox and monkeypox disease in 2019. Originally developed to address smallpox, it was also approved for an mpox indication by virtue of the vaccine challenge studies in animals having employed the monkeypox virus. Additionally, tecovirimat was made available during the mpox outbreak through a CDC investigational protocol and a National Institute of Allergy and Infectious Diseases clinical trial, as tecovirimat was not FDA approved for treating mpox (NLM, 2022; O'Laughlin et al., 2022). CDC distributed more than 80,000 bottles of oral tecovirimat and more than 13,000 vials of intravenous tecovirimat (Hruby, 2023). The investigational protocol may have allowed access but may also have created its own barriers, as the administrative burden of investigational new drug (IND) protocols is high and, some argue, may only be easily assumed by well-resourced health organizations (Cahill, 2023).

Multiple factors led to limited vaccine availability to initially respond to the 2022 mpox multi-country outbreak (Kota et al., 2023a). The stockpiling assumptions for MVA-BN were based on smallpox scenarios with a focus on accidental and deliberate release. BARDA had funded the advanced development of MVA-BN for its use as a smallpox preventive in immuno-compromised persons, and acquired it for the SNS via Project BioShield. While the stockpile had originally held 20 million doses of MVA-BN for use in a smallpox outbreak, most of those had expired, leaving the SNS in possession of 1.4 million filled doses (Chaplin, 2023). Of these, 372,000 doses were held in a Bavarian Nordic warehouse in Denmark and were ready to ship, but HHS was reportedly slow to request the full number of available doses, while 786,000 more doses met FDA inspection delays at the Danish facility before they could be shipped (LaFraniere et al., 2022).[2] Most of the supply owned by the U.S. government was available in bulk frozen product—as much as 15 million dose equivalents—but this could not be quickly formulated into individual thawed doses.

In addition to initial bottlenecks in providing MVA-BN at scale, demand for the this vaccine to contain mpox was not an anticipated SNS planning scenario. As the sole stockpile of vaccines approved for mpox, SNS leadership needed to evaluate releasing material potentially to the detriment of national security purposes. During the first year of the 2022 mpox outbreak, 748,329 first doses of MVA-BN were administered in the United States (Kota et al., 2023a). As of April 2023—nearly the 1-year mark of the outbreak—about two-thirds of vaccine-eligible people were still not vaccinated. Though vaccination rates were higher among ethnic minority groups, mpox incidence was also higher among these groups. Additionally, vaccination rates among Black and Hispanic males were disproportionate to incidence, revealing a higher unmet need for vaccination in these groups (Kota et al., 2023b).

---

[2] This information regarding vaccine shipments was modified after release of the prepublication version of the report in order to be more consistent with the cited reference.

Global Cooperation

COVID-19 and the ongoing mpox outbreak demonstrated the speed with which biothreats occurring anywhere in the world can impact and overwhelm national medical and public health response systems—which is a sobering reality of today's global interconnected supply chains and populations as well as the ongoing lack of health system capacities and coordination in health emergencies. The COVID-19 pandemic highlighted the critical importance of global preparedness and international cooperation for equitable and effective responses to emerging infectious diseases. Similarly, the mpox outbreak underscored the need for rapid detection, containment, and coordinated response efforts locally to mitigate impacts at national, regional, and global scales. The shortfalls of the global MCM enterprise during these events to ensure equitable access to MCMs in the United States and globally, along with enduring concerns about public acceptability of countermeasures, hindered disease containment around the globe. In response to these lessons, WHO Member States established an intergovernmental negotiating body "to draft and negotiate a WHO convention, agreement, or other international instrument on pandemic prevention, preparedness, and response" (WHO, 2023).

Strengthening smallpox MCM preparedness requires prioritizing proactive global cooperation, information sharing, capacity building, and joint research efforts to effectively respond to an outbreak anywhere in the world. COVID-19 underscored how effective response cannot be assumed based on better preparedness (IPPPR, 2021). Since eradication, understandably, most countries have not stockpiled smallpox MCMs or the other resources needed to respond to an outbreak. Therefore, global cooperation, information sharing and sharing financial and facility support for research to develop smallpox MCMs would be an essential first step in improving global readiness to a smallpox event.

While this report focuses primarily on smallpox MCMs developed for use in the United States and maintained in the SNS, WHO Member States may benefit from, and in some cases depend on, U.S. donations of smallpox vaccines or other MCMs. Moreover, in the event of a non-U.S. smallpox outbreak, the United States would derive significant health and security benefits by assisting other countries in the response to prevent the outbreak from spreading internationally.

SMALLPOX EMERGENCE AND RESPONSE CONSIDERATIONS

The needs of an MCM response will depend on the scale and circumstances of a potential smallpox outbreak. Since the eradication of naturally occurring smallpox, preparedness plans have focused on the potential for an accidental or deliberate reintroduction of smallpox. These scenarios have been based on intelligence of foreign bioweapons programs and the potential for breaches in biosafety at official laboratories with ongoing variola virus research (Bipartisan Commission on Biodefense, 2024; Department of State, 2023). Several factors have implications for the types, quantities, and potential utility of MCMs to contain smallpox. A few of the factors the committee considered in their deliberations are listed in Box 1-2. However, this summary is not exhaustive, and a comprehensive threat assessment, accompanied by scenario-based planning, as discussed in Chapter 4, is crucial to determining the appropriate assumptions. Chapter 3 further expands on specific factors that may influence readiness and response.

The relative utility of MCMs for immediate and long-term containment after a smallpox event can also help inform planning. As noted in past scenario-based assessments of smallpox readiness, most of the same activities are needed in terms of planning before an event, however, there will be greater variability in the resources and activities required for response (IOM, 2005). The demands that various smallpox containment strategies will place on the MCM enterprise in an outbreak will need to be considered in planning. For example, Biggs and Littlejohn describe a "hierarchy of MCMs against emerging biological threats" where higher-order MCMs (e.g., vaccines) offer increased protection with less frequency of administration over a longer period of time and therefore may be considered more effective for protection, compared with lower-order MCMs (e.g., personal protective equipment [PPE]) (Biggs and Littlejohn, 2022).[3] Figure 1-2 presents a conceptual hierarchy of MCMs, adapted for the smallpox readiness and response context. Though the use of PPE is important to infection prevention and included in the figure, the utility of this MCM was not considered in scope for this report.

OVERARCHING CONCLUSION

Based on the evidence and findings on the implications of the U.S. smallpox MCM enterprise for potential global smallpox events, the committee drew the following overarching conclusion:

> In a smallpox event, the U.S. readiness and response posture will be significantly affected by the ability of other countries around the world to adequately detect smallpox and contain transmission. Given global interdependence and global supply chains, supporting MCM capacities and capabilities internationally (i.e., a global MCM platform) will improve security against biothreats in the United States.

---

[3] Biggs describes durability as referring to the scope of protection, duration, and frequency to be administered, while resource use is inversely related due to the investment needed to sustain protection.

BOX 1-2
Summary of Factors Considered by the Committee

The committee considered the following in their evaluation of the state of smallpox MCM readiness:

Environmental Resurrection/Mutation and Engineered Variola or Variola-Like Virus
The effectiveness of MCMs developed to detect, prevent, and treat smallpox have been established based on their use against eradicated strains of variola. While current smallpox MCMs are cross-reactive for other orthopoxviruses and are expected to provide some benefit against a novel orthopoxvirus, MCMs are likely to be less effective against a variola or variola-like strain that is deliberately engineered to evade current vaccines and antivirals.

Accidental and Deliberate Release of Variola Virus
Differences in exposure scenarios would impact the speed with which an immediate response would need to be scaled. In the event of a laboratory accident or discovery of unofficial samples, direct and prolonged close contact would be needed for person-to-person transmission to continue to second- and third-generation smallpox cases. If these types of incidents occur in the United States, it would require reporting to CDC, with a response conducted in collaboration with WHO.

A deliberate release, as in the case of bioterrorism, would depend on the delivery system used. A bioterrorism attack in a populous area would expose a larger than normal number of individuals to smallpox simultaneously. MCM effectiveness would depend on the strain of the virus used in the attack and response measures would need to be accelerated immediately to protect the public. Additionally, exposure to a higher viral dose could result in more severe presentations of smallpox, such as hemorrhagic disease, and greater viral shedding, morbidity, and mortality as has been observed with mpox in an animal model (Hutson et al., 2010).

Delivery could also occur via an individual who has self-inoculated with variola or variola-like virus with the intent to spread disease, assuming the virus is viable through the delivery system over a defined period.

Geographic Scope
In the event of an accidental or deliberate smallpox outbreak, initial cases could be localized or across multiple locations. Regardless of the geographical scope, a smallpox outbreak of any size would likely constitute an international emergency, as it may indicate a nefarious actor with the motivation and capability to conduct subsequent attacks.

Immediate Containment and Post-Event
The MCMs needed and strategies used to implement them are likely to shift based on the goals of the response. The immediate response goals would be to contain transmission and mitigate morbidity and mortality. Longer term prevention would be implemented through a pre-exposure MCM program. Overall response

BOX 1-2 Continued

strategies would need to consider pre-exposure or post-exposure vaccination and antiviral prophylaxis and treatment (Chapter 2).

MCM Development, Storage, and Administration (Chapters 2 and 3)
- **Commercial manufacturing capability** – Currently, there is a lack of commercial market for smallpox MCMs and insufficient capacity to scale MCM production in the event of a large-scale smallpox event. The commercialization of cross-protective orthopoxvirus MCMs and emerging biotechnologies could provide capabilities to respond and deploy smallpox MCMs on demand, when and where needed.
- **Future development and utility of MCMs** – New MCM technologies could present opportunities to develop more effective MCMs against smallpox. A strategic approach to assessing the utility of newer MCMs, coupled with a research agenda, could improve readiness.
- **Storage requirements** – Lyophilized second-generation vaccines have continued to meet potency requirements, while the stability of third-generation vaccines will need to be assessed over time. Potency testing and shelf-life extension requirements are important to maintaining the utility of all stockpiled assets.
- **Distribution requirements** – The scope and nature of the outbreak would determine the conditions under which distribution for vaccines and therapeutics may differ.
- **Vaccine administration** – Multiple puncture (or scarification) is the technique used to administer first- and second-generation vaccines using a bifurcated needle. These vaccines produce a localized reaction (i.e., "take") and carry safety concerns in some populations.

MCM Utility and Acceptance (Chapters 2 and 3)
- **Vaccine and therapeutic safety and applicability** – Different vaccines and therapeutics are more appropriate for certain sub-populations due to (a) contraindications, (b) risk of exposure to smallpox, (c) containment strategy.
- **Acceptance and willingness to use MCMs** (Chapter 3) – Despite vaccine and therapeutics benefits, including protection from severe disease and reduced transmission, it is expected that segments of the public will refuse vaccination, testing, and/or therapeutics. These factors can be influenced by the willingness of state, tribal, local, and territorial governments to request and distribute MCMs, individual experiences in accessing MCMs, and concerns over safety or adverse reactions. Therefore, actual demand for MCMs may be lower than the forecasted needs.

SOURCES: Costantino et al., 2018; Gaudioso et al., 2011; Hutson, et al. 2010; Sloane, 2023.

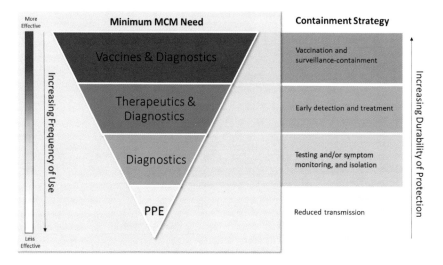

FIGURE 1-2 Minimum smallpox MCM needs according to containment strategy.
SOURCE: Adapted from Biggs and Littlejohn (2022).

REFERENCES

ASPR (Administration for Strategic Preparedness and Response). n.d. *SNS products: Vaccines and treatment available for use in the mpox response.* https://aspr.hhs.gov/SNS/Pages/Mpox.aspx (accessed November 30, 2023).

Behnam, M., A. Dey, T. Gambell, and V. Talwar. 2020. *COVID-19. Overcoming supply shortages for diagnostic testing.* McKinsey & Company. https://www.mckinsey.com/~/media/McKinsey/Industries/Pharmaceuticals%20and%20Medical%20Products/Our%20Insights/COVID%2019%20Overcoming%20supply%20shortages%20for%20diagnostic%20testing/COVID-19-Overcoming-supply-shortages-for-diagnostic-testing-vF2.pdf (accessed March 1, 2024).

Biggs, A. T., and L. F. Littlejohn. 2022. A hierarchy of medical countermeasures against biological threats. *Military Medicine* 187(7–8):830–836.

BioSpace. 2004. *United States pledges 20 million doses of smallpox vaccine to global stockpile.* https://www.biospace.com/article/releases/-b-u-s-department-of-health-and-human-services-b-release-united-states-pledges-20-million-doses-of-smallpox-vaccine-to-global-stockpile (accessed February 23, 2024).

Bipartisan Commission on Biodefense. 2020 (November). *Diagnostics for biodefense: Flying blind with no plan to land.* Washington, DC: Bipartisan Commission on Biodefense. https://biodefensecommission.org/wp-content/uploads/2020/11/Diagnostics-Special-Focus_final11_031421.pdf (accessed April 25, 2024).

Bipartisan Commission on Biodefense. 2021 (March). *Biodefense in crisis: Immediate action needed to address national vulnerabilities.* Washington, DC: Bipartisan Commission on Biodefense. https://biodefensecommission.org/wp-content/uploads/2021/03/Indicators-Report_final7_070221_web.pdf (accessed April 25, 2024).

Bipartisan Commission on Biodefense. 2024. *Box the pox: Reducing the risk of smallpox and other orthopoxviruses.* Washington, DC: Bipartisan Commission on Biodefense. https://biodefensecommission.org/wp-content/uploads/2024/02/2024.02.20-Box-the-Pox.pdf (accessed February 22, 2024).

Branswell, H. 2022. Why COVID-19 vaccines are a freaking miracle. *STAT*, February 14. https://www.statnews.com/2022/02/14/why-covid-19-vaccines-are-a-freaking-miracle (accessed April 25, 2024).

Cahill, S. 2023. Lessons learned from the U.S. public health response to the 2022 mpox outbreak. *LGBT Health* 10(7):489–495.

CDC (U.S. Centers for Disease Control and Prevention). 2022. *Sonic Healthcare USA to begin monkeypox testing today, increasing nationwide testing capacity.* CDC Newsroom Release, July 18. https://www.cdc.gov/media/releases/2022/s0718-sonic-monkeypox-testing.html (accessed February 29, 2024).

CDC. 2023. *Review of the shortcomings of CDC's first COVID-19 test and recommendations for the policies, practices, and systems to mitigate future issues.* https://stacks.cdc.gov/view/cdc/126876 (accessed March 3, 2024).

Chaplin, P. 2023. Smallpox medical countermeasures. Presentation at Meeting 3 of the Committee on Current State of Research, Development, and Stockpiling of Smallpox MCMs of the National Academies. December 14. https://www.nationalacademies.org/event/41411_12-2023_meeting-3-of-the-committee-on-the-current-state-of-research-development-and-stockpiling-of-smallpox-medical-countermeasures (accessed February 23, 2024).

CIDRAP (Center for Infectious Disease Research and Policy). 2004. *U.S. pledges smallpox vaccine for world stockpile.* https://www.cidrap.umn.edu/smallpox/us-pledges-smallpox-vaccine-world-stockpile (accessed January 26, 2024).

Costantino, V., M. P. Kunasekaran, A. A. Chughtai, and C. R. MacIntyre. 2018. How valid are assumptions about re-emerging smallpox? A systematic review of parameters used in smallpox mathematical models. *Military Medicine* 183(7–8):e200–e207.

Craven, J. 2021. Will anti-vaxxers take the new COVID treatment pills? *Slate*, November 23.

Department of State. 2023. *Adherence to and compliance with arms control, nonproliferation, and disarmament agreements and commitments.* Washington, DC: Department of State. https://www.state.gov/wp-content/uploads/2024/01/APR23-2023-Treaty-Compliance-Report.pdf (accessed March 1, 2024).

Facher, L. 2022. Some Americans are hesitant about COVID vaccines. But they're all-in on unproven treatments. *STAT*, January 27. https://www.statnews.com/2022/01/27/some-americans-are-hesitant-about-covid-vaccines-but-theyre-all-in-on-unproven-treatments (accessed April 25, 2024).

FDA (U.S. Food and Drug Administration). 2020a. *Coronavirus (COVID-19) update: FDA authorizes first COVID-19 test for self-testing at home.* https://www.fda.gov/news-events/press-announcements/coronavirus-covid-19-update-fda-authorizes-first-covid-19-test-self-testing-home (accessed February 29, 2024).

FDA. 2020b. *FDA approves first treatment for COVID-19.* https://www.fda.gov/news-events/press-announcements/fda-approves-first-treatment-covid-19 (accessed February 29, 2024).

FDA. 2023a. *Animal rule information.* https://www.fda.gov/emergency-preparedness-and-response/mcm-regulatory-science/animal-rule-information (accessed February 2, 2024).

FDA. 2023b. *Monkeypox (mpox) and medical devices.* https://www.fda.gov/medical-devices/emergency-situations-medical-devices/monkeypox-mpox-and-medical-devices#Laboratories (accessed February 6, 2024).

Fenner, F., D. A. Henderson, I. Arita, Z. Jezek, and I. D. Ladnyi. 1988. *Smallpox and its eradication.* Geneva: World Health Organization.

Gaudioso, J., T. Brooks, K. Furukawa, and D. Lavanchy. 2011. Likelihood of smallpox recurrence. *Journal of Bioterrorism & Biodefense* 2(2):106.

Gerald, N. 2023. Smallpox medical countermeasures. Presentation at Meeting 3 of the Committee on Current State of Research, Development, and Stockpiling of Smallpox MCMs of the National Academies. December 14. https://www.nationalacademies.org/event/41411_12-2023_meeting-3-of-the-committee-on-the-current-state-of-research-development-and-stockpiling-of-smallpox-medical-countermeasures (accessed February 23, 2024).

Henderson, D. A. 2009. *Smallpox: The death of a disease: The inside story of eradicating a worldwide killer.* Amherst, NY: Prometheus Books.

Hill, L., S. Artiga, A. Rouw, and J. Kates. 2022. *How equitable is access to COVID-19 treatments?* KFF, June 23. https://www.kff.org/coronavirus-covid-19/issue-brief/how-equitable-is-access-to-covid-19-treatments (accessed April 3, 2024).

Hruby, D. 2023. TPOXX: An orthopox antiviral. Presentation at Meeting 3 of the Committee on Current State of Research, Development, and Stockpiling of Smallpox MCMs of the National Academies. December 14. https://www.nationalacademies.org/event/41411_12-2023_meeting-3-of-the-committee-on-the-current-state-of-research-development-and-stockpiling-of-smallpox-medical-countermeasures (accessed February 23, 2024).

Hutson, C. L., D. S. Carroll, J. Self, S. Weiss, C. M. Hughes, Z. Braden, V. A. Olson, S. K. Smith, K. L. Karem, R. L. Regnery, and I. K. Damon. 2010. Dosage comparison of Congo Basin and West African strains of monkeypox virus using a prairie dog animal model of systemic orthopoxvirus disease. *Virology* 402(1):72–82.

IOM (Institute of Medicine). 2005. *The smallpox vaccination program: Public health in an age of terrorism.* Washington, DC: The National Academies Press.

IOM. 2009. *Live variola virus: Considerations for continuing research:* Washington, DC: The National Academies Press.

IPPPR (Independent Panel for Pandemic Preparedness and Response). 2021. *COVID-19: Make it the last pandemic.* https://theindependentpanel.org/wp-content/uploads/2021/05/COVID-19-Make-it-the-Last-Pandemic_final.pdf (accessed February 23, 2024).

Karem, K. L., M. Reynolds, Z. Braden, G. Lou, N. Bernard, J. Patton, and I. K. Damon. 2005. Characterization of acute-phase humoral immunity to monkeypox: Use of immunoglobulin M enzyme-linked immunosorbent assay for detection of monkeypox infection during the 2003 North American outbreak. *Clinical and Diagnostic Laboratory Immunology* 12(7):867–872.

Korch, G. W. 2016. *Product life cycle management and the PHEMCE: Lessons.* https://www.medical-countermeasures.gov/media/36964/21_korch_phemce.pdf (accessed April 25, 2024).

Kota, K. K., H. Chesson, J. Hong, C. Zelaya, I. H. Spicknall, A. P. Riser, E. Hurley, D. W. Currie, R. R. Lash, N. Carnes, J. Concepcion-Acevedo, S. Ellington, E. D. Belay, and J. Mermin. 2023a. Progress toward equitable mpox vaccination coverage: A shortfall analysis—United States, May 2022–April 2023. *Morbidity and Mortality Weekly Report* 72(23):627–632.

Kota, K. K., J. Hong, C. Zelaya, A. P. Riser, A. Rodriguez, D. L. Weller, I. H. Spicknall, J. L. Kriss, F. Lee, P. Boersma, E. Hurley, P. Hicks, C. Wilkins, H. Chesson, J. Concepción-Acevedo, S. Ellington, E. Belay, and J. Mermin. 2023b. Racial and ethnic disparities in mpox cases and vaccination among adult males—United States, May–December 2022. *Morbidity and Mortality Weekly Report* 72(15):398–403.

Kuiken, T., and F. Gottron. 2023. *The Strategic National Stockpile: Overview and issues for Congress.* Congressional Research Services R47400. https://crsreports.congress.gov/product/pdf/R/R47400 (accessed February 23, 2024).

LaFraniere, S., N. Weiland, and J. Goldtsein. 2022. U.S. could have had many more doses of monkeypox vaccine this year. *The New York Times,* August 3.

Leggat-Barr, K., N. Goldman, and F. Uchikoshi. 2021. COVID-19 risk factors and mortality among Native Americans. *Demographic Research* 45(39):1185–1218.

Lewis, R. 2023. Variola virus research: Overview of main activities and use of live virus. Presentation at Meeting 2 of the Committee on Current State of Research, Development, and Stockpiling of Smallpox MCMs of the National Academies. December 1. https://www.nationalacademies.org/event/41410_12-2023_meeting-2-of-the-committee-on-the-current-state-of-research-development-and-stockpiling-of-smallpox-medical-countermeasures (accessed February 23, 2024).

Lewis, T. 2022. U.S. monkeypox response has been woefully inadequate, experts say. *Scientific American,* July 14. https://www.scientificamerican.com/article/monkeypox-testing-and-vaccination-in-u-s-have-been-vastly-inadequate-experts-say1 (accessed February 23, 2024).

Li, Y., V. A. Olson, T. Laue, M. T. Laker, and I. K. Damon. 2006. Detection of monkeypox virus with real-time PCR assays. *Journal of Clinical Virology* 36(3):194–203.

Li, Y., H. Zhao, K. Wilkins, C. Hughes, and I. K. Damon. 2010. Real-time PCR assays for the specific detection of monkeypox virus West African and Congo Basin strain DNA. *Journal of Virological Methods* 169(1):223–227.

Magesh, S., D. John, W. T. Li, Y. Li, A. Mattingly-app, S. Jain, E. Y. Chang, and W. M. Ongkeko. 2021. Disparities in COVID-19 outcomes by race, ethnicity, and socioeconomic status: A systematic review and meta-analysis. *JAMA Network Open* 4(11):e2134147.

Murphy, S. J., L. W. Samson, and B. D. Sommers. 2022. *COVID-19 antivirals utilization: Geographic and demographic patterns of treatment in 2022.* Department of Health and Human Services Office of the Assistant Secretary for Planning and Evaluation, December 23.

Maxmen, A. 2020. Thousands of coronavirus tests are going unused in U.S. labs. *Nature* 580(7803):312–313.

NASEM (National Academies of Sciences, Engineering, and Medicine). 2021. *Ensuring an effective Public Health Emergency Medical Countermeasures Enterprise.* Washington, DC: The National Academies Press.

NIBIB (National Institute of Biomedical Imaging and Bioengineering). 2022. *RADx initiative: Bioengineering for COVID-19 at unprecedented speed and scale.* https://www.nibib.nih.gov/about-nibib/directors-corner/corner-posts/radx-initiative-bioengineering-covid-19-unprecedented-speed-and-scale (accessed March 2, 2024).

NIBIB. n.d. *Independent Test Assessment Program (ITAP).* https://www.nibib.nih.gov/covid-19/radx-tech-program/ITAP (accessed December 19, 2023).

NLM (National Library of Medicine). 2022. *Study of tecovirimat for human monkeypox virus (STOMP).* https://clinicaltrials.gov/study/NCT05534984?term=NCT05534984&rank=1 (accessed December 13, 2023).

O'Donnell, C., and A. Abouleneim. 2021. U.S. testing struggles to keep up with Omicron. *Reuters.* https://www.reuters.com/world/us/us-testing-struggles-keep-up-with-omicron-2021-12-22 (accessed March 1, 2024).

O'Laughlin, K., F. A. Tobolowsky, R. Elmor, R. Overton, S. M. O'Connor, I. K. Damon, B. W. Petersen, A. K. Rao, K. Chatham-Stephens, P. Yu, and Y. Yu. 2022. Clinical use of tecovirimat (TPOXX) for treatment of monkeypox under an investigational new drug protocol—United States, May–August 2022. *Morbidity and Mortality Weekly Report* 71(37):1190–1195.

Our World in Data. 2020. *COVID-19: Daily tests vs. daily new confirmed cases per million.* https://ourworldindata.org/grapher/covid-19-daily-tests-vs-daily-new-confirmed-cases-per-million?time=earliest..2020-02-25&country=ARE~KOR~RUS (accessed December 6, 2023).

Robinson, P. C., D. F. L. Liew, H. L. Tanner, J. R. Grainger, R. A. Dwek, R. B. Reisler, L. Steinman, M. Feldmann, L. P. Ho, T. Hussell, P. Moss, D. Richards, and N. Zitzmann. 2022. COVID-19 therapeutics: Challenges and directions for the future. *Proceedings of the National Academy of Sciences* 119(15):e2119893119.

Sloane, M. 2023. USG needs and factors for consideration. Presentation at Meeting 3 of the Committee on Current State of Research, Development, and Stockpiling of Smallpox MCMs of the National Academies. December 14. https://www.nationalacademies.org/event/41411_12-2023_meeting-3-of-the-committee-on-the-current-state-of-research-development-and-stockpiling-of-smallpox-medical-countermeasures (accessed February 23, 2024).

Smyth, J., C. Gilbert, and K. Stacey. 2022. America's COVID testing system buckles under weight of Omicron surge. *Financial Times.* https://ft.com/content/8602434b-3366-4075-b9a0-51cea67b-5cbe (accessed March 1, 2024).

Suran, M. 2022. Expanding monkeypox testing. *JAMA* 328(4):321.

WHO (World Health Organization). 1980. *Global smallpox eradication.* Geneva: World Health Organization.

WHO. 1986. Committee on orthopoxvirus infections: Report of the fourth meeting. *Weekly Epidemiological Record (Relevé épidémiologique hebdomadaire)* 61(38):289–293. https://iris.who.int/bitstream/handle/10665/225977/WER6138_289-293.PDF?sequence=1 (accessed February 23, 2024).

WHO. 1996. WHA49.10 *Smallpox eradication—destruction of variola virus stocks.* https://iris.who.int/bitstream/handle/10665/179420/WHA49_R10_eng.pdf?sequence=1 (accessed February 23, 2024).

WHO. 1999. *WHA52.10 smallpox eradication: Destruction of variola virus stocks.* https://iris.who.int/bitstream/handle/10665/79354/e10.pdf (accessed February 23, 2024).

WHO. 2002. *Global public health response to natural occurrence, accidental release or deliberate use of biological and chemical agents or radionuclear material that affect health.* https://apps.who.int/gb/archive/pdf_files/WHA55/ewha5516.pdf (accessed February 23, 2024).

WHO. 2007. *WHA60.1 smallpox eradication: Destruction of variola virus stocks.* https://iris.who.int/bitstream/handle/10665/22569/A60_R1-en.pdf?sequence=1 (accessed January 26, 2024).

WHO. 2016. *Post-eradication.* https://www.who.int/news-room/feature-stories/detail/post-eradication (accessed January 26, 2024).

WHO. 2017. *Operational framework for the deployment of the World Health Organization Smallpox Vaccine Emergency Stockpile in response to a smallpox event.* Geneva: World Health Organization. https://www.who.int/publications/i/item/WHO-WHE-IHM-2017-14 (accessed February 23, 2024).

WHO. 2023. *Building a resilient world together: The intergovernmental negotiating body for pandemic preparedness.* Geneva: World Health Organization.

WHO. 2024. *154th session of the executive board, provisional agenda item 18—Smallpox eradication: Destruction of variola virus stocks (January 2, 2024).* https://apps.who.int/gb/ebwha/pdf_files/EB154/B154_20-en.pdf (accessed February 23, 2024).

Wolford, T., J. Sutton, and C. N. Mangal. 2023. Laboratory responses to pandemic threats: Challenges, needs, and solutions. *Health Security* 21(S1):S56–S59.

Yamey, G., A. V. Diez Roux, J. Clark, and K. Abbasi. 2024. Pandemic lessons for the 2024 presidential election. *BMJ* 384:q150.

Zimmer, C. 2021. How the search for COVID-19 treatments faltered while vaccines sped ahead. *The New York Times*, September 28.

2

State of Smallpox Medical Countermeasures Readiness

"The eradication of smallpox occurred prior to the development of the majority of modern virological and molecular biological techniques. Therefore, there is a considerable amount that is not understood regarding how this solely human pathogen interacts with its host."

John Connor, in presentation to the committee
January 12, 2024, in reference to Olson and Shchelkunov (2003)

A variety of medical countermeasures (MCMs) have been developed to detect (diagnostics), prevent (vaccines), and treat (biological agents and antivirals) smallpox disease and transmission. This section summarizes the key characteristics of these assets—focusing on gaps and future opportunities, including emerging technologies. One fundamental lesson learned from COVID-19 and mpox emergencies is that research and development for new smallpox MCMs must not only consider the characteristics of the "product" but also must consider the ability to deploy at scale and ensure equitable access.

DIAGNOSTICS, DETECTION, AND SURVEILLANCE

The ability to rapidly detect and diagnose a potential case of smallpox is central to all containment strategies. In the United States, the primary strategy for containment involves vaccination coupled with surveillance (Henderson and Klepac, 2013; Petersen et al., 2015). Outside of environmental detection systems for smallpox, which operate in limited capacity, the early identification of a smallpox case is presumed likely to occur based on clinical suspicion of smallpox or a non-variola orthopoxvirus. Clinical suspicion of

41

smallpox would be followed by testing for variola virus, whereas continued clinical suspicion of a non-variola orthopoxvirus for which non-variola orthopoxvirus testing is negative would require follow-on testing for the variola virus itself. In the United States, testing would be conducted by a U.S. Centers for Disease Control and Prevention (CDC) Laboratory Response Network (LRN) laboratory, with CDC conducting confirmatory testing on any positive samples with further confirmatory testing at CDC for any initially variola virus–positive results (CDC, 2017b). As there are few practicing clinicians in the United States who have ever seen a person with smallpox, delays in diagnosis based on clinical suspicion are likely.

Testing Options and Utility

U.S. diagnostic testing options to confirm smallpox rely on a variola-specific assay approved by the U.S. Food and Drug Administration (FDA) in 2017. The FDA-approved Variola Virus Nucleic Acid-Based Detection Assay is indicated for "individuals presenting with pustular or vesicular rash illness or other signs and symptoms of Variola virus infection" (FDA, 2024b). This is the only variola-specific assay available in the United States outside of CDC. This test is available at some LRN laboratories as part of a clinical testing algorithm, with positive results requiring confirmatory testing at CDC via single-gene PCR (polymerase chain reaction) testing and subsequent confirmation via additional genomic testing (Hutchins et al., 2008).

Electron microscopy (EM) or cell culture may additionally be used to provide evidence of an orthopoxvirus or indicate infectivity, respectively, however these techniques alone are not diagnostic for smallpox (CDC, 2016, 2017b). However, negative-stain EM is less sensitive than PCR, there are few laboratories with expertise in this technique, and its use may be limited to additional corroborative testing. Tissue and pathology sample evaluation with immunohistochemical staining is another diagnostic option.

Gaps and System Pain Points

Concerns with Clinical Recognition Capability

The identification of smallpox cases requires clinical recognition. While clinician awareness of orthopoxvirus infections has increased in the United States due to the multi-country mpox outbreak, the rise of mpox could also obscure an outbreak of smallpox or another novel orthopoxvirus. A recent report describing the first fatal case of Alaskapox infection showed that over 6 weeks had passed between the patient's first reported symptoms and a laboratory confirmation of Alaskapoxvirus (Rogers et al., 2024). Additionally, due to the low positive predictive value of smallpox diagnostics in the absence of known disease,[1] the identification of suspected and probable smallpox cases relies on a patient first meeting a clinical case definition prior to testing (CDC, 2017a). These factors could hamper immediate identification of a smallpox outbreak, especially if case definitions are not appropriate or the initial cases present in an atypical fashion. For example, case definitions used in early days of the COVID-19 pandemic were overly strict by emphasizing travel to Wuhan, China (Suthar et al., 2022). Historically, early waves of the smallpox outbreak in ex-Yugoslavia in 1972 where the index case had an atypical presentation without scarring (Ristanovic et al., 2016).

During the 2022 mpox outbreak, once CDC and FDA began supporting orthopoxvirus testing in five commercial laboratory companies, clinicians preferred to use these laboratories over the public health laboratories of the LRN due to more streamlined patient data requirements and perhaps the perception of a more rapid availability of actionable results initially made possible by higher throughput testing capabilities at commercial laboratories (APHL, 2023). The addition of commercial laboratories also increased testing capacity significantly (CIDRAP, 2022). Better understanding of data needs and decision-making and distribution timelines could have implications for laboratory planning for an evolving smallpox outbreak, especially around clinician education, the distribution and ubiquity of laboratory-based tests, and, critically for the questions posed to this committee, the level of investment by the Biomedical Advanced Research and Development Authority (BARDA) in point-of-care diagnostics for the U.S. Strategic National Stockpile (SNS) and for routine use.

Limited Availability of Diagnostic Assays

Diagnostic assays for variola are available only at select LRN laboratories, largely due to biosafety considerations, and only as part of a clinical testing algorithm. The approach to only test at LRNs with confirmation at CDC may affect testing turnaround times during a larger outbreak. The current algorithm was designed for the detection of initial cases in the absence of endemic disease, but planning for laboratory capacity should include strategies for both immediate response and long-term scenarios where greater demand for testing arises. Greater availability of reliable laboratory-based tests for smallpox may enhance the nation's ability to rapidly respond to a smallpox outbreak, although easier access to testing would also presumably increase the frequency of false positive tests, making effective clinician education even more important. Additionally, expanding the number

---

[1] For rare diseases, positive tests are more likely to be wrong than when the disease is commonly occurring.

of sites that can conduct both variola-specific and orthopoxvirus diagnostic testing would require concurrent improvements to laboratory biosafety and management of potential associated biosecurity concerns.

Lack of FDA-Cleared Serological Assays

FDA-cleared serological assays for smallpox have not been developed, and protein-based tests are still being explored. Lateral-flow assay tests so far do not offer high enough sensitivity to reliably detect orthopoxviruses and need further confirmation against clinical specimens (Ulaeto et al., 2022).

Future Opportunities and Emerging Diagnostic Technologies

The 2022 multi-country mpox outbreak spurred the development of numerous mpox and pan-orthopoxvirus diagnostics, which are now at various stages along research, development, or regulatory approval pathways. These include assets based on loop-mediated isothermal amplification (LAMP) technology, rapid diagnostics, serological assays, and a GeneXpert test; their potential effectiveness for smallpox has not been assessed. Numerous non-variola tests (e.g., mpox and pan-orthopox) developed by academic and commercial developers and used with FDA enforcement discretion policies could play an important role in a future smallpox event (FDA, 2023c). Many of these tests have been described in the literature, including real-time PCR assays used for mpox and an enzyme-linked immunosorbent assay (ELISA), for both IgG and IgM, used on subjects from Wisconsin, which was the epicenter of the 2003 U.S. mpox outbreak (Hammarlund et al., 2005; Karem et al., 2005; Y. Li et al., 2006). Any work which uses live variola virus to validate smallpox diagnostics must also be approved by the World Health Organization (WHO) Advisory Committee on Variola Virus Research (ACVVR). The lack of a sustained commercial market has likely deterred ongoing commitments for commercial assay developers.

Develop Point-of-Care and Point-of-Need Tests

Point-of-care (POC)/point-of-need (PON) tests for smallpox remain elusive.[2] LAMP diagnostic assays, a relatively recent development in nucleic acid amplification, were developed and improved on during the 2022 mpox response and might be useful for POC testing in the event of a smallpox

---

[2] POC test: clinical lab testing conducted close to the site of patient care where treatment will be provided. PON test: that provided at a location where an ill/exposed person can go to be tested and, if positive, go to a care site if needed. The PON test may be much more widely accessible than a POC test.

outbreak, but they would need further real-world evaluation against the outbreak-causing strain (Z. Li et al., 2023). After 2022 FDA issued Emergency Use Authorizations (EUAs) for additional testing platforms, such as the Cepheid mpox assay (FDA, 2023d). Such advancements could aid in the development of future variola diagnostics particularly if developed for smaller multiplex platforms and equipment used within the clinical settings. These and other POC assays using protein or antigen-detection may be useful for initial testing to inform isolation and other public health decisions (Lewis, 2023; Meyer et al., 2020). Additionally, as has been noted with other high consequence pathogens, POC tests may also have a role to play in early evaluation of patients in resource scarce settings as well as use in mobile testing (Bhadelia, 2015; Castillo-Leon et al., 2021; Dhillon et al., 2015). Deployment of POC testing would need to be accompanied with patient and provider education about the limitations and use cases for these technologies, in partnership with public health authorities (Kost, 2021). Given the high public health concern regarding smallpox cases, rapid diagnostics aimed at the consumer are unlikely to have a role in most smallpox outbreaks.

Expand PCR Assays and Platforms

As discussed in Chapter 1, a limiting factor to expanding testing during the 2022 mpox multi-country outbreak was a lack of diverse testing assays and platforms at the beginning of the outbreak. Expansion of PCR assays and platforms, such as the development of pan-orthopoxvirus assays or variola-specific assays on a variety of platforms, could help reduce dependence on a single product, potentially reducing testing bottlenecks and increasing test accessibility. Additionally, platforms that can perform testing at different biosafety levels and at field sites would be useful in improving global access to testing.

The Non-Variola Orthopoxvirus Real-Time PCR Primer and Probe Set is a pan-orthopox DNA test approved by FDA in 2022 to qualitatively detect all orthopoxviruses, except variola and Alaskapox viruses (FDA, 2024a; Rogers et al., 2024). The test cannot identify the specific non-variola orthopoxvirus that may be causing disease. This test was used for laboratory diagnosis during the 2003 U.S. mpox outbreak response and has been used extensively since 2022. Additional PCR assays tailored for a range of platforms can increase the diversity of products available during an outbreak and improve the ability to bring testing closer to the patients, while avoiding testing and manufacturing bottlenecks.

In a potential outbreak, it is likely that the first patients evaluated for smallpox will already have rash illness and will have been infectious to others for several days prior to recognition. PCR testing can produce reliable results rapidly and is commonly used on lesion-based samples including exudate, roofs from lesions, and lesion crusts (CDC, 2017b). During the mpox response, nucleic acid testing also found mpox in oral and naso-pharyngeal specimens, rectal tissue, semen, saliva, urine, and feces (Peiró-Mestres et al., 2022). Although the pathogenic mechanism for this observation may differ between clade IIb monkeypoxvirus infection and variola virus infection, this compares to reports of finding variola virus in saliva, conjunctiva, and urine in patients with hemorrhagic smallpox (Sarkar et al., 1973). Expanded availability of PCR testing in other sample types might allow for earlier disease identification and containment, making it the preferred method for variola testing. Identification of biomarkers for presymptomatic detection of smallpox patients and improvements to methodologies for automatic extraction methods for PCR testing could also be useful.

Antibody testing utility is low, as for all acute illnesses, due to the time lag in antibody development, which results in poor prospects for early detection. There could be utility in using antibody titers as correlates of protection in those with prior vaccination and to understand population-level exposures and immunity to smallpox (Moss, 2011).

Genomic and Environmental Surveillance

While this report is primarily concerned with clinical screening and diagnostic tools that can support smallpox readiness and response, population-level and environmental surveillance tools and systems can also support preparedness and may rely on the same kinds of technologies and technological advances critical to clinical assay development. Genomic and environmental surveillance can be used to monitor shifts in circulating poxvirus genomes; information about such shifts may support predictions of increased or decreased virulence or transmission. Genomic surveillance during an outbreak supported by bioinformatics software, such as Nextstrain, can also provide critical feedback on real-time viral evolution (Hadfield et al., 2018).

The environmental detection program, BioWatch, operated by the Department of Homeland Security, is designed to provide early alerts concerning aerosolized pathogens of concern by sampling air in strategic locations throughout the United States and coupling this with laboratory testing of the samples (IOM and NRC, 2011). Wastewater surveillance systems for disease detection were built in response to COVID-19 and were used for the detection of mpox, mostly using PCR-based tests (Oghuan et al., 2023). Future expansion of wastewater surveillance to aircraft-based networks could potentially act as an early warning system (J. Li et al., 2023). Metagenomic approaches to surveillance hold the potential to improve detection of pathogens that may not be normally suspected in a non-endemic area (Ko et al., 2022;

Sharma et al., 2023). Additionally, viral genomics and phylogenetic analyses have become important parts of public health investigations and are critical to stay ahead of pathogen evolution for emerging and priority pathogens and would be a critical component in the public health toolbox in case of a smallpox outbreak (Di Paola et al., 2020; Saravanan et al., 2022).

Conclusions on Diagnostics, Detection, and Surveillance

(2-1) Tests that can more accurately detect smallpox and other orthopoxviruses than those available today are needed; efforts should focus on (1) adapting multiplex nucleic acid assays for new platforms and field settings, (2) developing forward-deployed (POC/PON) assays to enhance equitable access to tests, including protein or antigen-based tests to rapidly test and isolate infected patients, (3) identifying FDA-approved serologic assays to assess individual and population levels of immunity against smallpox and history of related exposures, (4) validating nucleic acid testing using a variety of clinical samples, (5) developing different categories of laboratory tests for different biosafety levels, and (6) supporting a global network of laboratories to detect, diagnose, and conduct surveillance in humans and the environment.

VACCINES

As observed in the early phases of the smallpox eradication program, robust surveillance and containment strategies implemented concurrently with ring vaccination—the targeted vaccination of contacts of cases, contacts of contacts, and others at high risk of exposure—was paramount to mitigating or eliminating human-to-human transmission (IOM, 2002; Lane, 2006). A ring-vaccination-based containment approach was effective to eradicate naturally occurring smallpox due to the long incubation period of smallpox (and mpox) in humans. This made ring vaccination for smallpox and mpox, even after exposure, epidemiologically, clinically, and economically efficient at mitigating or eliminating illness and subsequent transmission compared with mass vaccination (Foege, 2011; Sah et al., 2022). Ring vaccination is also still recommended by both WHO and CDC as the first-line response strategy for a smallpox outbreak (CDC, 2019b; WHO, 2023). However, both CDC and the WHO Strategic Advisory Group of Experts on Immunization (SAGE) note that the scale of vaccination (from ring vaccination to mass vaccination) may be determined based on risk and the outbreak characteristics and the groups needing vaccinated.

For a bioterrorist attack, particularly one occurring in a populous city, mass vaccination post-event, or following an immediate response to contain spread, has also been discussed as an effective strategy. Models and simulation exercises from the early 2000s highlighted logistical challenges and the inability for ring vaccination to be scaled rapidly enough post-event to be effective (Bicknell, 2002; Kaplan et al., 2002). In the early 2000s, preemptive mass vaccination also carried greater risk of adverse events, compared to the limited benefits afforded when the threat of a bioterrorist attack remained small (Fauci, 2002).

Uncertainties in the expected need to provide smallpox vaccine for the entire population makes it reasonable to plan for scenarios where the entire population needs vaccination. However, planning considerations would need to reflect more recent population characteristics and increasing potential for *de novo* synthesis or deliberate engineering to cause a smallpox event (see Chapter 2).

The Institute of Medicine's (IOM's) previous reports *Live Variola Virus: Considerations for Continuing Research* (2009) includes a detailed summary of the history of smallpox vaccine development—from early vaccine development to post-eradication era—and describes how the development of smallpox vaccines has progressed in major phases (first-, second-, third-generation) (IOM, 2009). The effectiveness of vaccines developed post-eradication to prevent disease, transmission, hospitalization, or death in the event of a smallpox or novel orthopoxvirus outbreak will remain unknown due to the inability to test vaccine effectiveness against active smallpox infections. Licensure for newer vaccines must rely on non-inferiority data for immunogenicity and protection in animal challenge models compared with first-generation or second-generation smallpox vaccines. This challenge also highlights the importance of being able to rapidly deploy adaptable clinical trials if an outbreak does occur (see Chapter 4 for more details on research readiness).

Vaccine Options and Utility

Currently, the U.S. stockpile maintains three different smallpox vaccines, all of which are based on vaccinia virus: two types of live, replicating virus vaccines; and an attenuated live, non-replicating vaccine as well as ancillary supplies for their administration (Table 2-1). The two types of replication-competent vaccinia virus vaccines in the SNS are Smallpox (Vaccinia) Vaccine, live (ACAM2000), which is a second-generation vaccine based on the first-generation vaccine Dryvax, and Aventis Pasteur Smallpox Vaccine (APSV), or WetVax, which is a first-generation vaccine (i.e., liquid formulation of calf-lymph-origin vaccinia virus vaccine) that was manufactured from 1956 to 1957 and has been maintained at –20°C (CDC, 2019a; Petersen et al., 2015). APSV is intended to be used only after ACAM2000 is exhausted, its potency is verified, and if approved for use in a smallpox emergency under an appropriate regulatory mechanism, specifically an EUA or an investigational new drug (IND) application (CDC, 2022). Live, replicating vaccinia virus vaccines are expected to be used to contain

TABLE 2-1 Summary of Smallpox Vaccines in the U.S. Strategic National Stockpile

Product Name	Characteristics	Approved Usage	Formulation and Storage
APSV (Wetvax)	1st generation Live, replicating vaccinia virus, NYCBOH-derived strain.	• Emergency Use Authorization (EUA)/ Investigational New Drug (IND) for smallpox. • 1 dose regimen. • Multiple contraindications, especially for those who have immunocompromising, skin, or heart conditions. Contraindicated for those with serious allergy to a vaccine component.	Formulation contains live vaccinia virus in 50% glycerol, 0.4% phenol, 0.00017% Brilliant Green, and frozen at –20°C.
ACAM2000	2nd generation Live, replicating vaccinia virus, NYCBOH-derived strain.	• FDA licensed for prevention of smallpox in all age groups for those at high-risk for smallpox infection. • 1 dose regimen. • Multiple contraindications, especially for those who have immunocompromising, skin, or heart conditions. Contraindicated for those with serious allergy to a vaccine component.	Lyophilized (1×10^8 pfu/ml when reconstituted), diluent is 50% Glycerin USP and 0.25% phenol USP in water, stored at –20°C.
MVA-BN (Imvamune, Imvanex, JYNNEOS)	3rd generation Live, non-replicating vaccinia virus, MVA strain.	• FDA licensed for smallpox and Mpox in adults 18 and older. • 2 dose regimen, 4 weeks apart. • Relatively few contraindications. Safely administered to individuals with immunocompromising, skin, or heart conditions. Contraindicated for those with serious allergy to a vaccine component.	Liquid, 10mM Tris, 140mM sodium chloride, host cell DNA (≤20mcg) and protein (≤500mcg), benzonase (≤0.0025mcg), gentamicin (≤0.400mcg), and ciprofloxacin (≤20.005mcg), stored frozen at –25°C to –15°C.

SOURCES: Adams (2023); FDA (2021a, 2022); Petersen et al. (2015)

transmission following a deliberate or accidental release of smallpox, as well as for a post-event vaccination program (Petersen et al., 2015). These vaccines are also the predominant type among the current cached vaccine assets and are intended to be available in sufficient quantity for the entire U.S. population (Adams, 2023).

Non-replicating vaccines were acquired more recently to provide an alternative for individuals contraindicated to receiving replicating smallpox vaccine. Modified vaccinia Ankara vaccine-Bavarian Nordic (MVA-BN), marketed in the United States as JYNNEOS and elsewhere as Imvamune, or Imvanex, is a third-generation live, non-replicating vaccine developed in collaboration with the U.S. government. MVA-BN was developed post-eradication, and therefore not tested in a smallpox endemic setting. Studies using first-generation vaccine as a challenge, found that MVA-BN vaccination prior to vaccination with Dryvax decreased the primary cutaneous reaction and decreased the time to healing, suggesting that MVA-BN would be protective against smallpox (Frey et al., 2007; Parrino et al., 2007; Pittman et al., 2019; Seaman et al., 2010). A phase 3 trial also observed fewer adverse events among those who received two doses of MVA-BN compared to individuals who only received Dryvax (Pittman et al., 2019). The Department of Health and Human Services (HHS) has procured MVA-BN for the SNS at smaller volumes than first- and second-generation vaccines and intends to use it primarily for populations with contraindications to those vaccines (Wolfe, 2023). Additionally, the utility of MVA-BN in a ring vaccination strategy for immediate containment has not been demonstrated due to the use of a two-dose regimen. In 2023 the Advisory Committee on Immunization Practices updated recommendations for the use of MVA-BN in adults at risk for mpox, and the Strategic Advisory Group of Experts on Immunization recommended that WHO add MVA-BN to its stockpiles and review protocols for smallpox (CDC, 2023a; WHO, 2023).

The level of humoral antibody needed to provide protection against smallpox following vaccination is unknown. Data from eradication efforts suggested that a neutralizing antibody titer of more than 1:20 or more than 1:32 resulted in some level of protection against symptomatic illness (Mack et al., 1972). Currently licensed vaccines could not, for ethical reasons, include human vaccine efficacy trials. Therefore, vaccines were licensed using neutralizing antibody titer equivalence. The true efficacy as well as the duration of immunity is unknown, as was the case during the pre-eradication era. It is believed that persons who had past exposure to variola virus or received only primary immunization would have lifelong protection from fatal infection (Taub et al., 2008).

Box 2-1 provides an overview of the characteristics of first-, second-, and third-generation vaccines as well a placeholder for potential fourth-generation vaccines, which are expected to provide improvements in safety, efficacy, administration, or other key characteristics.

BOX 2-1
Smallpox Vaccine Summary and Terminology

First Generation (e.g., Dryvax, APSV)

- Live vaccinia virus vaccines developed before and during the smallpox eradication effort.
- Typically produced by infecting large animals and collecting, purifying, and lyophilizing the lymph exudate.
- Administered percutaneously using a bifurcated needle as a single dose.
- Characteristic "take," or scar develops at vaccination site.
- Estimated high efficacy rates (typically >91%).
- Side effects and adverse events vary by virus strain.
- Multiple contraindications, especially for those who are immunocompromised or have skin or heart conditions.

Second Generation (e.g., ACAM2000)

- Live vaccinia virus vaccines developed using clonal derivatives of 1st generation vaccines (Dryvax).
- Produced in mammalian cell culture or in embryonated eggs using good manufacturing practice (GMP) methods.
- Administered percutaneously using a bifurcated needle as a single dose.
- Characteristic "take," or scar develops at vaccination site.
- Similar immunogenicity to 1st generation vaccines.
- No efficacy data available against smallpox (developed after eradication).
- Fewer side effects and adverse events than 1st generation vaccines.
- Multiple contraindications, especially for those who are immunocompromised or have skin or heart conditions.

Third Generation (e.g., MVA-BN)

- Vaccines containing highly attenuated live vaccine or non-replicating strains of vaccinia virus.
- Produced in mammalian cell culture, embryonated eggs, or Chicken Embryo Fibroblast cells (e.g., for MVA-BN specifically) using GMP methods.
- Administered by injection.
- MVA-based formulations require two doses, at 0 and 4 weeks, do not induce formation of a "take."
- Immunogenicity after all doses (i.e., non-inferior to 1st and 2nd generation vaccines).
- No efficacy data available against smallpox (developed after eradication).
- Far fewer side-effects and adverse events than 1st and 2nd generation vaccines.
- Relatively few contraindications. Safely administered to individuals with HIV, cancer patients, organ transplant recipients, and individuals on immunosuppressive therapies.

continued

BOX 2-1 Continued

Fourth Generation (none currently licensed or stockpiled; in clinical development only)

*   Potential subunit or nucleic acid vaccines (protein, peptide, mRNA) lacking replicating vaccinia virus.

SOURCES: CDC (2023c); Kennedy and Gregory (2023); Petersen et al. (2015).

Gaps and Pain Points

Safety Concerns and Adverse Events

The safety profiles of ACAM2000 and APSV (Wetvax) are expected to be similar to Dryvax (first-generation vaccine), as both vaccines are based on the New York City Board of Health (NYCBOH) strain used in Dryvax (Petersen et al., 2015). Adverse events, though rare, can be severe and life-threatening (Table 2-2). Historical data indicate that first-generation vaccines were associated with at least 1 death per million primary vaccinations given, with the higher frequency of adverse events arising following primary vaccination and in younger children (Belongia and Naleway, 2003). It is important to note however that these data come from a period when smallpox vaccines were administered within the first months of life, knowledge of cell-mediated immunity was lacking, and some contraindications could not be accurately diagnosed in young infants. More recently, a voluntary smallpox vaccination program implemented in 2002 using second-generation vaccines among military personnel and civilians was discontinued by June 2003 due to cases of myo/pericarditis, concerns of viral shedding and risk of vaccinia infection to others, and at least three deaths (IOM, 2005).

CDC's clinical use guidelines for smallpox vaccine indicate that there are no absolute contraindications for a smallpox vaccination in a post-event setting but that there are certain "relative" contraindications due to the possibility of adverse events associated with certain conditions (Table 2-2). CDC developed its recommendations for smallpox use by weighing risk for smallpox infection, risk for an adverse event following vaccination, and benefit from vaccination (Petersen et al., 2015). Relative contraindications include atopic dermatitis (eczema), HIV infection (CD4 cell counts of 50–199 cells/mm^3), other immunocompromised states, and allergies to the vaccine or vaccine components. The adverse events can range from generalized vaccinia, a rash resulting from spread of the replicating virus from the injection site, to myopericarditis and death. The rates of these events are variable and, in some cases, unknown (Table 2-2).

TABLE 2-2 Potential Adverse Events Associated with Smallpox Vaccination with Replicating Vaccine

Adverse Event	Description	Historical Risk of Complication
Auto-inoculation	Transfer of the virus from the injection site to another site on the body or to another individual. Lesions occur on new site with the same progression as the vaccine site. If transferred to the eye, vaccinia keratitis, corneal scarring, and blindness can occur.	0–1647 per million primary vaccinations 0–675.7 per million revaccinations
Bacterial infections	Bacterial infection of the vaccination site; typically, staphylococci or group A streptococci. Can be minimized by appropriate vaccine site care. Typically responds well to antimicrobials.	No historical frequency data reported.
Congenital vaccinia	Infection in utero can occur after vaccination of pregnant women. Exceptionally rare and results in stillbirth or death of the newborn shortly after birth.	~10–100 per million vaccinations
Death	Typically, due to post-vaccinal encephalitis (fatality rate = 25%), progressive vaccinia (fatality rate nearly 100% and eczema vaccinatum (10% before vaccinia immune globulin [VIG], 2% afterward).	Historically reported as 1–2 deaths per million primary vaccinations. Often in young children or those with unrecognized defects in T cell immunity.
Eczema vaccinatum	Large areas of the skin become covered in confluent lesions. Untreated, this can lead to systemic symptoms and septic shock. VIG treatment is effective if given within 1–2 days of symptom onset. This adverse event is seen in recipients with underlying skin conditions (eczema, atopic dermatitis) even without active disease.	8.1–96.8 per million primary vaccinations 0–13.5 per million revaccinations
Generalized vaccinia	Viremia and rash spreading from vaccination site or occurring elsewhere on the body. Most cases resolve without treatment. VIG can be used, as can treatment appropriate for known immune abnormalities.	20.8–387.1 per million primary vaccinations 0–9.0 per million revaccinations
Myopericarditis	Inflammation of the heart muscle or the pericardium/pericardial space. Can be accompanied by shortness of breath, chest discomfort, or pain. Symptoms occur 4–30 days after vaccination.	Not assumed to be vaccine-related and therefore not well documented during eradication era.

continued

TABLE 2-2 Continued

Adverse Event	Description	Historical Risk of Complication
		Post-eradication data from military populations indicate a rate of 80–160 cases per million primary vaccine recipients.
		Reports focusing on civilian populations have a higher rate ~500 cases per million vaccinees.
Non-infectious rashes (erythema multiforme)	Generalized rash occurring 1–2 weeks after vaccination. Most resolve spontaneously and can be managed by over-the-counter treatments. Rarely, they can result in hospitalization. Stevens-Johnson syndrome and death have also been reported.	51.5–164.6 per million primary vaccinations 2.1–10 per million revaccinations
Post-vaccinal encephalitis	Encephalitis occurs 1–2 weeks after vaccination, causing one or more of the following: headache, drowsiness, vomiting, muscular weakness, ataxia, paralysis, coma, convulsion. Has a fatality rate of 25%. In 50% of survivors, some degree of neurologic damage is present, which can be permanent. No known predictors of susceptibility markers. VIG is not effective.	1.5–176.5 per million primary vaccinees 0–2 per million re-vaccinees
Progressive vaccinia (disseminated vaccinia, vaccinia necrosum)	Characterized by a failure of vaccine site to heal, progressive spreading of the lesion in the absence of inflammation, viremia leading to additional lesions on distal sites that follow the same progressive spread. Believed to be a result of a defective or inadequate T cell response. Bacterial infection is common, and patients can suffer from toxic or septicemic shock. Treatment with VIG was used in the 1960s with partial success. Recently developed antiviral drugs (e.g., Cidofovir or ST-246) may be effective.	0–6.9 per million primary vaccinations 0–6 per million revaccinations

SOURCES: Aragón et al. (2003); Arness et al. (2004); Engler et al. (2015); Lane et al. (1969, 1970); Morgan et al. (2008); Murphy et al. (2003); Neff et al. (1967a,b); Ratner et al. (1970); Ryan et al. (2008); Tack et al. (2013).

Due to this potential for severe adverse events in certain immunocompromised persons, CDC recommends that people with relative contraindications be vaccinated with MVA-BN. Clinical trials involving healthy and high-risk populations, such as those with HIV infection, have reported no cases of myo-/pericarditis after vaccination with MVA-based vaccines, whereas myo-/pericarditis was observed with the use of first-and second-generation live smallpox vaccines (Overton et al., 2015; Zitzmann-Roth et al., 2015). The rates and severity of mostly mild, self-limiting common side effects (e.g., headache, fever, myalgia, regional lymphadenopathy) are broadly similar for MVA-BN and ACAM2000.

The main disadvantages of MVA-BN in a post-event setting are that it requires two injections given 4 weeks apart, and, unlike replicating vaccines, its real-world efficacy against smallpox is unknown and has been assessed only through animal models, serological endpoints, and non-inferiority studies. Vaccination campaigns using non-replicating MVA-BN to vaccinate persons at risk of mpox provide additional valuable data and demonstrate effectiveness rates for two doses ranging from 66 percent to 86 percent (Dalton et al., 2023; Deputy et al., 2023; Rosenberg et al., 2023). While MVA-BN is safe for immunocompromised persons and should provide protection for those at risk of eczema vaccinatum, effectiveness in severely immunodeficient populations is expected to be lower due to inability to mount an effective immune response after vaccination (CDC, 2023b). However, it is unknown whether an exposure dose–response or exposure based on differing modes of transmission (e.g., sexual contact related disease vs. other modes of mpox transmission) is associated with observed vaccine efficacy.

Reliance on the U.S. Strategic National Stockpile and Concerns with Manufacturing Capacity

Dependence on the SNS smallpox vaccine stockpile as the primary form of smallpox readiness has required that sufficient inventory be maintained to respond to a smallpox event where the entire U.S. population could potentially require vaccination. This explains, in part, the large proportion of spending that has gone to smallpox MCM. Under the current stockpiling strategy, ACAM2000 will be the primary vaccine used in a smallpox response scenario. While older second-generation vaccines in the SNS are thought to be quite stable, their potency is less well understood, and MVA-BN had been intended to be used for only a subset of the population. While quantities of stockpiled vaccine doses are not released publicly, research estimates put the U.S. immunocompromised population (the main population for which MVA-BN is intended) at approximately 15 percent of the population, more than 49 million people, rising to about 38 percent if their household contacts are included (Adams, 2023; Carlin et al., 2017).

Notably, this figure does not include the population with post-acute sequelae of SARS-CoV-2 (long COVID), who appear to have immune dysfunction following COVID-19 infection, though the committee found no evidence that such a state would be an absolute or relative contraindication to live smallpox vaccination (Phetsouphanh et al., 2022). The risks and benefits of live vaccine for the heterogeneous immunocompromised population must be weighed. Finally, a likely approach to contain a smallpox outbreak would be to use both vaccines and therapeutics. However, the potential interactions between vaccines and antivirals if used concomitantly are not well understood (Russo et al., 2020).

The choice to focus on stockpiling vaccines has been driven, in part, by limited production capacity, which makes it difficult to rapidly manufacture additional smallpox vaccine doses. Smallpox vaccines are not mass-market vaccines that are produced in a routine manner using widely available ingredients and common manufacturing processes. Ramping up the production of smallpox vaccines to meet a sudden demand would require procuring potentially limited raw materials and navigating multiple regulatory and safety hurdles.

Future Opportunities and Emerging Vaccine Technologies

Opportunities for newer vaccines include the development of those with fewer contraindications, broad protection, single-dose administration, and stable shelf-life. As noted by the WHO ACVVR, the development of "scalable less-reactogenic vaccines" with improved efficacy and durability of protection would be "essential for the control of an outbreak of smallpox in the current context, should it recur" (WHO, 2024). Research on fourth generation smallpox vaccines could explore potential subunit or nucleic acid vaccines (protein, peptide, mRNA) lacking replicating vaccinia virus.

Explore Innovative Vaccine Platforms

Safe and effective COVID-19 vaccines were made in under a year since the start of the pandemic due to decades of research on mRNA vaccines and U.S. government investment in mRNA platform technology (NIH, 2022). Smallpox vaccine development could benefit from investments in novel, rapid vaccine platforms such as mRNA, viral vectors, and protein nanoparticles. Like for most potential vaccine targets, mRNA technology may be a useful approach; however, the utility of this approach, specifically for orthopoxviruses remains uncertain. There is work underway evaluating novel mRNA constructs, however (Hou et al., 2023), and the National Institutes of Health (NIH) is supporting the development of mRNA-based vaccines for orthopoxviruses (Freyn et al., 2023; HHS, 2023). Modified vaccinia Ankara (MVA) has also shown utility as a vaccine vector for non-orthopoxvirus pathogens (e.g., HIV, malaria, Ebola, tuberculosis, MERS-CoV) as well as in oncolytic virotherapies (Lin et al., 2023; Orlova et al., 2022). While any vaccine using the MVA backbone would provide some protection against smallpox and other orthopoxviruses, the utility of recombinant MVA vaccines to contain a smallpox emergency is uncertain.

Develop Immunobridging Strategy

Development of an immunobridging strategy would be important to allow for useful cross-vaccine comparisons, especially as there is no way to effectively test a smallpox vaccine for efficacy against smallpox. This type of approach has been considered for COVID-19, filovirus as well as for seasonal influenza vaccines (Gruber et al., 2023; Khoury et al., 2023). Basic clinical trials for safety and immunogenicity can be accomplished through routine clinical development strategies along with relevant antecedent preclinical studies. Further work into the utility of fourth-generation vaccines that use multi-vaccine platforms and immunobridging strategies would allow for greater diversity in the vaccine products that are available. Diversification of MCM products in the SNS is highlighted in Chapter 4.

Conclusions on Vaccines

(2-2) Smallpox vaccines that have improved safety across different population subgroups and are available as a single dose would support faster and more effective response to contain smallpox and other orthopoxvirus outbreaks. The development of novel smallpox vaccines using multi-vaccine platforms (i.e., use common vaccine vectors, manufacturing ingredients, and processes) would improve the capacity for rapid vaccine production in response to a smallpox event and reduce the need for stockpiling in the SNS at current levels.

THERAPEUTICS

Initiated in the late 1990s, the initial approach to developing smallpox treatments was to screen small molecule compounds and further develop those that demonstrate activity across orthopoxviruses (OPXVs) (Baker et al., 2003). More recent efforts have evaluated anti-variola and anti-orthopoxvirus activity with a focus on biologics, such as monoclonal antibodies, antibody cocktails, and vaccinia immunoglobulin (VIG), as well as antivirals with distinct mechanisms of action (Martins, 2023). Table 2-3 presents a summary of smallpox antivirals with additional details on their mechanisms of action, indications, bioavailability, and storage.

TABLE 2-3 Summary of Smallpox Therapeutics in the U.S. Strategic National Stockpile

Product Name	Mechanism of Action	Indication	Bioavailability	Formulation and Storage

Tecovirimat (ST-246/TPOXX)	Orthopoxvirus-specific inhibition of viral spread from cell to cell by targeting p37, a major envelope protein required for envelopment and excretion of extracellular forms of the virus.	• Treatment of smallpox (FDA approved)
		 • Other uses for treatment of mpox under Investigational New Drug (IND), Expanded Access IND, Emergency IND (not FDA approved)
		   ○ STOMP/A5418 (Study of Tecovirimat for Human Mpox Virus)[a]
		   ○ STOMP sub-study of open label tecovirimat[b]
		   ○ STOMP sub-study: Tecovirimat for Orthopox Virus Exposure[c]
			• Oral formulation: 48% oral bioavailability with enhanced absorption when taken with food (DeLaurentis et al., 2022). The FDA approval is for oral administration within 30 minutes of a moderate-to high-fat meal. Maximum concentration is at 4 hours post oral dose.
			 • IV formulation: Max concentration at the end of recommended infusion given over 6 hours.
				Capsules stored in the original bottle at 20°C to 25°C (68°F to 77°F); excursions permitted 15°C to 30°C (59°F to 86°F).
				
				 Injection stored at 2°C to 8°C (36°F to 46°F).

				FDA had initially approved a shelf-life extension of tecovirimat injection from 24 months to 42 months for some lots (FDA, 2023b).

Brincidofovir (CMX001/ Tembexa)	Pro-drug of cidofovir[f]; following phosphorylation of the prodrug to the active form cidofovir diphosphate which targets the orthopoxvirus DNA polymerase, causing disruption of replication of the virus.	• Treatment of human smallpox infections only (FDA approved)
		 • Other uses[d] (EIND or EA IND):
		   ○ Study to Assess Brincidofovir Treatment of Serious Diseases or Conditions Caused by Double-Stranded DNA viruses[e] (phase 3 completed December 2022)
		   ○ Adenovirus in immuno-compromised persons: under clinical trial
			• The lipid modification of cidofovir that created this drug enhances its oral bioavailability in oral tablet and suspension formulations.
			 • The tablet has 13.4% bioavailability whereas the suspension has 16.8% bioavailability.
			 • Best absorption is when taken on an empty stomach or with a low-fat meal.
				Oral suspension—expiry 30 months from the date of manufacture when stored at 20°C to 25°C (68°F to 77°F) (FDA, 2021b).
				
				 Tablets—expiry 48 months from the date of manufacture when stored at 20°C to 25°C (68°F to 77°F).

| Vaccinia Immune Globulin Intravenous Human (VIGIV) (CNJ-016) | Passive immunity for individuals with complications to vaccinia virus following vaccination; exact mechanism of action is not known. | • Treatment of complications due to vaccinia vaccination (FDA approved) • Other uses (EA IND): Potential use of stockpiled VIGIV for treatment of orthopoxviruses in an outbreak | • Maximum concentration at 6,000 U/kg dose reached in 1.8 ±1.2 hours, and with 9,000 U/kg dose was reached at 2.6 ±2.4 hours after administration. • Available upon clinician request to CDC on case-by-case basis for intravenous administration. | Stored frozen at or below 5°F (≤ −15°C) or refrigerated at 36°F to 46°F (2°C to 8°C); if received frozen, use within 60 days of thawing at 36°F to 46°F (2°C to 8°C). |

NOTES: Cidofovir (Vistide), another antiviral not currently stockpiled, targets orthopoxvirus DNA polymerase, causing disruption of replication of the virus. The licensed indication is for cytomegalovirus (CMV) retinitis and does not have licensed indication for OPXV/VARV therapy. However, it can be used "off label." Cidofovir was used in therapy of mpox in those with compromised immune systems/uncontrolled HIV during the 2022–2023 multi-country outbreak, as this treatment was commercially available. Potential side effects include renal toxicity.

CDC = U.S. Centers for Disease Control and Prevention; EA = expanded access; EIND = emergency investigational new drug application; IND = investigational new drug application; OPXV = orthopoxvirus; VARV = variola virus.

[a] NIH/NIAID-sponsored: Phase 3 randomized, placebo-controlled, double-blind study to establish the efficacy of tecovirimat for the treatment of people with laboratory-confirmed or presumptive human monkeypox virus disease (HMPXV) [NCT05534984].

[b] Open label for pregnant or breastfeeding persons; those with severe immune suppression, significant skin conditions, or severe disease.

[c] For both mpox and smallpox for Department of Defense–affiliated personnel [NCT02080767].

[d] There are no registered clinical trials for brincidofovir at this time, could be used under EIND through CDC.

[e] Phase 3 trial completed 12/2022 with posted results [NCT01143181].

[f] Cidofovir was used in therapy of mpox in those with compromised immune systems/uncontrolled HIV during the 2022–2023 multi-country outbreak, as this treatment was commercially available.

SOURCES: Chan-Tack et al. (2021); Emergent BioSolutions Canada Inc. (2018); Gilead Sciences (2000); Grosenbach et al. (2011, 2018); Huston et al. (2023); Jordan et al. (2010); Merchlinsky et al. (2019); Yang et al. (2005).

Potential smallpox therapeutics can only be tested in vitro against variola virus or by using nonhuman animal models or surrogate viruses (e.g., non-variola virus). Such testing data, coupled with pharmacokinetic and safety data in humans, has allowed for FDA approval of tecovirimat and brincidofovir under the Animal Rule pathway (FDA, 2023a). Additionally, in many studies assessing the efficacy of antivirals against mpox in small animals, therapeutics were administered prior to the onset of rash illness (Hutson and Damon, 2010). More recent efforts have looked at therapeutic efficacy in nonhuman primates when initiated after rash onset following exposure to mpox (Russo et al., 2018). Because clinical guidelines rely on the presentation of rash illness to collect specimens for testing and to identify probable smallpox cases, the effectiveness of these therapeutics against the most likely early case presentations (i.e., people with a smallpox rash) is uncertain. Experience with the mpox outbreak revealed that those with severe immunosuppression required extended courses of treatment, often using multiple therapeutics (Pinnetti et al., 2023).

Therapeutics Options and Utility

Smallpox antiviral research and development efforts to date have resulted in two antiviral agents that are FDA approved for the treatment of human smallpox in adult and pediatric patients: tecovirimat and brincidofovir (CDC, 2023d,e). These products have different mechanisms of action and oral bioavailability (see Table 2-3). Both tecovirimat and brincidofovir were approved under the Animal Rule and must be requested from the SNS, as neither is commercially available. Tecovirimat is efficacious as a post-exposure therapeutic treatment of orthopoxvirus, specifically mpox, and its utility as a pre-exposure prophylaxis in high-risk humans is likely following observed therapeutic benefits in nonhuman primates evaluated in a prelesional and postlesional setting (Mucker et al., 2013). Cidofovir, a commercially available drug approved by FDA in 1996 for the treatment of AIDS-related cytomegalovirus (CMV) retinitis, was also used "off label" to treat mpox in immunocompromised individuals during the 2022 multi-country mpox outbreak (Siegrist and Sassine, 2023). Cidofovir has a more severe side effect profile than brincidofovir and is only recommended when the latter is not readily available.

Gaps and Pain Points

Lack of Diverse Antivirals

The two approved antivirals have independent mechanisms of action and are not antagonistic of each other. While brincidofovir slows DNA synthesis, tecovirimat inhibits membrane protein p37 that is essential for formation of an enveloped virus, so both could be used in combination (Siegrist, 2023). However, the effectiveness and utility of combination therapies to improve treatment efficacy and reduce the potential of anti-viral resistance are yet to be determined (P. Li et al., 2023). Periodic evaluation of compound libraries may ultimately yield additional promising therapeutics. Additionally, it would be ideal to have antivirals that act upon different stages of the virus lifecycle, (e.g., targeting specific virion components or other steps of viral infection) to mitigate the potential for antiviral resistance (Delaune and Iseni, 2020). Finding drugs that target and kill only the virus without damaging host cells is also a challenge because viruses use the host's cell to replicate (Kausar et al., 2021). In addition to considering the mechanisms of action, diverse modes of antiviral administration might provide increased protection. In one study, aerosolized cidofovir was found to protect mice against an otherwise lethal challenge of aerosolized cowpox virus (Bray and Roy, 2004). A similar approach could be possible with aerosolized brincidofovir as well.

Concerns with Antiviral Resistance and Adverse Events

Antiviral resistance is a significant concern for the current antivirals. Stepwise resistance to cidofovir is known to occur when treating CMV, with moderate resistance with single mutations and a higher level of resistance with multiple mutations (Siegrist and Sassine, 2023). Notably, cidofovir-resistant virus is less virulent than wild type (CDV-sensitive) virus. Whether this would occur in the setting of monkeypox (MPXV) or VARV is unknown. With tecovirimat and brincidofovir, single amino acid resistance mutations have been observed, with questionable impacts on viral fitness (Foster et al., 2017; Smith et al., 2023).

Adverse events, such as serious renal toxicity, have been observed during treatment of CMV retinitis infections with cidofovir (Skiest et al., 1999). Additionally, intravenous tecovirimat is not recommended for patients with severe renal impairment (CDC, 2023d).

Future Opportunities and Emerging Therapeutic Technologies

Research and development efforts in the past 10 years have often focused on re-purposing non-vaccine biologics and antibody-derived therapeutics:

- **Vaccinia immune globulin intravenous (VIGIV)** is a polyclonal antibody therapy and FDA-licensed biological agent (since 2005) for the treatment or modification of complications resulting from vaccinia smallpox vaccination (CDC, 2023c). There is potential to repurpose this biologic for treatment of orthopoxviruses in an outbreak, however VIGIV has not been considered an effective standalone therapeutic for smallpox (Jahrling 2011). In response to the 2022 multi-country outbreak, expanded access for VIGIV was provided through an Investigational New Drug (IND) Application to treat mpox infection in adults and children in concert with small molecule compounds; however, data on efficacy are limited (Gilchuk et al., 2016).

- **BFI-753** (Biofactura), a two-antibody cocktail to treat smallpox, is in late preclinical development, with an anticipated IND application submission in 2025 (Martins, 2023).
- Preclinical studies on potential therapeutics targeting cellular proteins or systems required for the virus lifecycle, such as **imatinib mesylate** (Gleevec®), have not progressed past early-stage research and development efforts, as concerns remain about imatinib's potential for treating smallpox (Ananthula et al., 2018; IOM, 2009; Reeves et al., 2005, 2011). For example, animal model benefit required continuous pump infusion, indicating challenges with administration.
- **ST-357** (Siga Technologies), a smallpox antiviral with a mechanism of action distinct from tecovirimat and brincidofovir that targets conserved domains in orthopoxviruses, and which is undergoing testing in animal models (Hruby, 2023).
- **NIOCH-14** is a derivative of tricyclodicarboxylic acid and a precursor of tecovirimat developed and tested in the Russian Federation (ClinicalTrials.gov, 2023; Delaune and Iseni, 2020). In animal models (i.e., an Institute of Cancer Research mouse model and marmoset model using MPXV challenge), NIOCH-14 demonstrated equal efficacy to tecovirimat and purportedly is easier to produce (Delaune and Iseni, 2020; Mazurkov et al., 2016).
- Most recently, a **potential for custom designed antivirals** for orthopoxviruses has been demonstrated using CRISPR technologies in *in vitro* studies (Siegrist et al., 2020)

Conclusion on Therapeutics

(2-3) To treat smallpox, the following would be advantageous to develop in order to supplement the therapeutic options currently approved and stockpiled in the SNS (1) new, safer antivirals with different and diverse targets, mechanisms of action, and routes of administration that minimize damage to host cells and have a high barrier to the development of resistance; (2) combination antiviral treatments and treatments based on novel technologies and platforms (e.g., genome editing, non-conventional targets, etc.); (3) Vaccinia immune globulin intravenous (VIGIV) repurposed as part of combination therapy; (4) diverse options for non-vaccine biologics including monoclonal antibodies and antibody cocktails.

(2-4) Most mpox therapeutics were developed because of investments in small-pox therapeutics, resulting in products found to have activity against mpox. Direct investment in developing therapeutics targeting circulating orthopox-viruses could similarly benefit smallpox therapeutic preparedness and could likely have more immediate utility and potentially achieve commercial viability.

OVERARCHING CONCLUSION

Based on the evidence and findings on the current state of smallpox MCMs, the committee drew the following overarching conclusion:

The COVID-19 pandemic revealed weaknesses in the ability for the nation's public health and health care systems to rapidly and flexibly adapt the emergency response to an unfamiliar pathogen; whereas the 2022 mpox outbreak tested existing MCMs developed primarily for smallpox to contain a less lethal orthopoxvirus. The lessons learned from both emergencies call for strengthening the nation's laboratory response systems and further development of point-of-care diagnostics and genomics surveillance capabilities. Additionally, safer, single-dose vaccines and a diverse set of therapeutic options against smallpox would improve the U.S. readiness and response posture for immediate containment and long-term protection in a smallpox emergency.

REFERENCES

Adams, S. A. 2023. Strategic National Stockpile smallpox medical countermeasures overview. Presentation at Meeting 3 of the Committee on Current State of Research, Development, and Stockpiling of Smallpox MCMs of the National Academies. December 14. https://www.nationalacademies.org/event/41411_12-2023_meeting-3-of-the-committee-on-the-current-state-of-research-development-and-stockpiling-of-smallpox-medical-countermeasures (accessed February 23, 2024).

APHL (Association of Public Health Laboratories). 2023. *The need for LRN modernization through the lens of an outbreak.* https://www.aphl.org/aboutAPHL/publications/lab-matters/Pages/The-Need-for-LRN-Modernization.aspx (accessed March 1, 2024).

Ananthula, H. K., S. Parker, E. Touchette, R. M. Buller, G. Patel, D. Kalman, J. S. Salzer, N. Gallardo-Romero, V. Olson, I. K. Damon, T. Moir-Savitz, L. Sallans, M. H. Werner, C. M. Sherwin, and P. B. Desai. 2018. Preclinical pharmacokinetic evaluation to facilitate repurposing of tyrosine kinase inhibitors nilotinib and imatinib as antiviral agents. *BMC Pharmacology and Toxicology* 19(1):80.

Aragón, T. J., S. Ulrich, S. Fernyak, and G. W. Rutherford. 2003. Risks of serious complications and death from smallpox vaccination: A systematic review of the United States experience, 1963–1968. *BMC Public Health* 3:26.

Arness, M. K., R. E. Eckart, S. S. Love, J. E. Atwood, T. S. Wells, R. J. Engler, L. C. Collins, S. L. Ludwig, J. R. Riddle, and J. D. Grabenstein. 2004. Myopericarditis following smallpox vaccination. *American Journal of Epidemiology* 160(7):642–651.

Baker, R. O., M. Bray, and J. W. Huggins. 2003. Potential antiviral therapeutics for smallpox, monkeypox and other orthopoxvirus infections. *Antiviral Research* 57(1–2):13–23.

Belongia, E. A., and A. L. Naleway. 2003. Smallpox vaccine: The good, the bad, and the ugly. *Clinical Medicine & Research* 1(2):87–92.

Bhadelia, N. 2015. Rapid diagnostics for Ebola in emergency settings. *The Lancet* 386(9996):833–835.

Bicknell, W. J. 2002. The case for voluntary smallpox vaccination. *New England Journal of Medicine* 346(17):1323–1325.

Bray, M., and C. J. Roy. 2004. Antiviral prophylaxis of smallpox. *Journal of Antimicrobial Chemotherapy* 54(1):1–5.

Carlin, E. P., N. Giller, and R. Katz. 2017. Estimating the size of the U.S. population at risk of severe adverse events from replicating smallpox vaccine. *Public Health Nursing* 34(3):200–209.

Castillo-Leon, J., R. Trebbien, J. J. Castillo, and W. E. Svendsen. 2021. Commercially available rapid diagnostic tests for the detection of high priority pathogens: Status and challenges. *Analyst* 146:3750–3776.

CDC (U.S. Centers for Disease Control and Prevention). 2016. *Negative staining electron microscope protocol for rash illness.* https://www.cdc.gov/smallpox/lab-personnel/specimen-collection/negative-stain.html (accessed February 26, 2024).

CDC. 2017a. *Specimen collection and transport guidelines for suspect smallpox cases.* https://www.cdc.gov/smallpox/lab-personnel/specimen-collection/specimen-collection-transport.html (accessed February 6, 2024).

CDC. 2017b. *Smallpox: For clinicians—Diagnosis & evaluation.* https://www.cdc.gov/smallpox/clinicians/diagnosis-evaluation.html (accessed January 11, 2024).

CDC. 2019a. *Appendix A: Aventis Pasteur Smallpox Vaccine (APSV).* Youtube.com. https://www.youtube.com/watch?v=wIJU4DXEztA&t=1s (accessed February 23, 2024).

CDC. 2019b. *Smallpox: Vaccination strategies.* https://www.cdc.gov/smallpox/bioterrorism-response-planning/public-health/vaccination-strategies.html (accessed December 22, 2023).

CDC. 2022. *Smallpox: Vaccines.* https://www.cdc.gov/smallpox/clinicians/vaccines.html (accessed January 30, 2024).

CDC. 2023a. *ACIP recommendations: mpox vaccines.* https://www.cdc.gov/vaccines/acip/recommendations.html (accessed February 12, 2024).

CDC. 2023b. *Clinical considerations for treatment and prophylaxis of mpox infection in people who are immunocompromised.* https://www.cdc.gov/poxvirus/mpox/clinicians/people-with-HIV.html (accessed March 4, 2024).

CDC. 2023c. *Clinical treatment.* https://www.cdc.gov/poxvirus/mpox/clinicians/treatment.html (accessed February 6, 2024).

CDC. 2023d. *Guidance for tecovirimat use.* https://www.cdc.gov/vaccines/acip/recommendations.html (accessed February 12, 2024).

CDC. 2023e. *Treatment information for healthcare professionals.* https://www.cdc.gov/poxvirus/mpox/clinicians/treatment.html (accessed February 6, 2024).

Chan-Tack, K., P. Harrington, T. Bensman, S. Y. Choi, E. Donaldson, J. O'Rear, D. McMillan, L. Myers, M. Seaton, H. Ghantous, Y. Cao, T. Valappil, D. Birnkrant, and K. Struble. 2021. Benefit–risk assessment for brincidofovir for the treatment of smallpox: U.S. Food and Drug Administration's evaluation. *Antiviral Research* 195:105182.

CIDRAP (Center for Infectious Disease Research and Policy). 2022. *U.S. allows commercial labs to test for monkeypox.* https://www.cidrap.umn.edu/us-allows-commercial-labs-test-monkeypox (accessed March 1, 2024).

ClinicalTrials.gov. 2023. *Study of the safety, tolerability, pharmacokinetics of NIOCH-14 in volunteers aged 18–50 years.* https://clinicaltrials.gov/study/NCT05976100 (accessed February 6, 2024).

Dalton, A. F., A. O. Diallo, A. N. Chard, D. L. Moulia, N. P. Deputy, A. Fothergill, I. Kracalik, C. W. Wegner, T. M. Markus, P. Pathela, W. L. Still, S. Hawkins, A. T. Mangla, N. Ravi, E. Licherdell, A. Britton, R. Lynfield, M. Sutton, A. P. Hansen, G. S. Betancourt, J. V. Rowlands, S. J. Chai, R. Fisher, P. Danza, M. Farley, J. Zipprich, G. Prahl, K. A. Wendel, L. Niccolai, J. L. Castilho, D. C. Payne, A. C. Cohn, and L. R. Feldstein. 2023. Estimated effectiveness of JYNNEOS vaccine in preventing mpox: A multijurisdictional case–control study—United States, August 19, 2022–March 31, 2023. *Morbidity and Mortality Weekly Report* 72(20):553–558.

Delaune, D., and F. Iseni. 2020. Drug development against smallpox: Present and future. *Antimicrobial Agents and Chemotherapy* 64(4):e01683-19.

DeLaurentis, C. E., J. Kiser, and J. Zucker. 2022. New perspectives on antimicrobial agents: Tecovirimat for treatment of human monkeypox virus. *Antimicrobial Agents and Chemotherapy* 66(12):e0122622.

Deputy, N. P., J. Deckert, A. N. Chard, N. Sandberg, D. L. Moulia, E. Barkley, A. F. Dalton, C. Sweet, A. C. Cohn, D. R. Little, A. L. Cohen, D. Sandmann, D. C. Payne, J. L. Gerhart, and L. R. Feldstein. 2023. Vaccine effectiveness of JYNNEOS against mpox disease in the United States. *New England Journal of Medicine* 388(26):2434–2443.

Dhillon, R. S., D. Srikrishna, R. F. Garry, and G. Chowell. 2015. Ebola control: Rapid diagnostic testing. *The Lancet Infectious Diseases* 15(2):147–148.

Di Paola, N., M. Sanchez-Lockhart, X. Zeng, J. H. Kuhn, and G. Palacios. 2020. Viral genomics in Ebola virus research. *Nature Reviews Microbiology* 18(7):365–378.

Emergent BioSolutions Canada Inc. 2018. *Product monograph including patient medication information CNJ-016™*. https://www.emergentbiosolutions.com/wp-content/uploads/2022/01/VIGIV-Canada-Monograph-English.pdf (accessed February 23, 2024).

Engler, R. J., M. R. Nelson, L. C. Collins, Jr., C. Spooner, B. A. Hemann, B. T. Gibbs, J. E. Atwood, R. S. Howard, A. S. Chang, and D. L. Cruser. 2015. A prospective study of the incidence of myocarditis/pericarditis and new onset cardiac symptoms following smallpox and influenza vaccination. *PLOS One* 10(3):e0118283.

Fauci, A. S. 2002. Smallpox vaccination policy—the need for dialogue. *New England Journal of Medicine* 346(17):1319–1320.

FDA (U.S. Food and Drug Administration). 2021a. *JYNNEOS package insert*. https://www.fda.gov/media/131078/download (accessed March 4, 2024).

FDA. 2021b. *NDA approval–Animal efficacy Tembexa (brincidofovir)*. Edited by U.S. FDA. https://www.accessdata.fda.gov/drugsatfda_docs/appletter/2021/214460Origs000,214461Orig1s000ltr.pdf (accessed February 26, 2024).

FDA. 2022. *ACAM2000 (smallpox vaccine) questions and answers*. https://www.fda.gov/vaccines-blood-biologics/vaccines/acam2000-smallpox-vaccine-questions-and-answers (accessed March 3, 2024).

FDA. 2023a. *Animal rule information*. https://www.fda.gov/emergency-preparedness-and-response/mcm-regulatory-science/animal-rule-information (accessed February 2, 2024).

FDA. 2023b. *FDA mpox response*. https://www.fda.gov/emergency-preparedness-and-response/mcm-issues/fda-mpox-response (accessed February 6, 2024).

FDA. 2023c. *Monkeypox (mpox) and medical devices*. https://www.fda.gov/medical-devices/emergency-situations-medical-devices/monkeypox-mpox-and-medical-devices#Laboratories (accessed February 6, 2024).

FDA. 2023d. *Xpert mpox letter of authorization*. https://www.fda.gov/media/165317/download (accessed February 23, 2024).

FDA. 2024a. *Product classification: Non-variola orthopoxvirus real-time PCR primer and probe set*. https://www.accessdata.fda.gov/scripts/cdrh/cfdocs/cfpcd/classification.cfm?id=PBK (accessed January 17, 2024).

FDA. 2024b. *Product classification: Variola virus nucleic acid-based detection assay*. https://www.accessdata.fda.gov/scripts/cdrh/cfdocs/cfpcd/classification.cfm?id=PRA (accessed January 17, 2024).

Foege, W. 2011. Lessons and innovations from the West and Central African smallpox eradication program. *Vaccine* 29(Suppl 4):D10–D12.

Foster, S. A., S. Parker, and R. Lanier. 2017. The role of brincidofovir in preparation for a potential smallpox outbreak. *Viruses* 9(11):320.

Frey, S. E., F. K. Newman, J. S. Kennedy, V. Sobek, F. A. Ennis, H. Hill, L. K. Yan, P. Chaplin, J. Vollmar, B. R. Chaitman, and R. B. Belshe. 2007. Clinical and immunologic responses to multiple doses of imvamune (modified vaccinia Ankara) followed by Dryvax challenge. *Vaccine* 25(51):8562–8573.

Freyn, A. W., C. Atyeo, P. L. Earl, J. L. Americo, G. Chuang, H. Natarajan, T. R. Frey, J. G. Gall, J. I. Moliva, R. Hunegnaw, G. A. Arunkumar, C. O. Ogega, A. Nasir, G. Santos, R. H. Levin, A. Meni, P. A. Jorquera, H. Bennet, J. A. Johnson, M. A. Durney, G. Stewart-Jones, J. W. Hooper, T. M. Colpitts, G. Alter, N. J. Sullivan, A. Carfi, and B. Moss. 2023. An mpox virus mRNA-lipid nanoparticle vaccine confers protection against lethal orthopoxviral challenge. *Science Translational Medicine* 15(716):eadg3540.

Gilchuk, I., P. Gilchuk, G. Sapparapu, R. Lampley, V. Singh, N. Kose, D. L. Blum, L. J. Hughes, P. S. Satheshkumar, M. B. Townsend, A. V. Kondas, Z. Reed, Z. Weiner, V. A. Olson, E. Hammarlund, H. P. Raue, M. K. Slifka, J. C. Slaughter, B. S. Graham, K. M. Edwards, R. J. Eisenberg, G. H. Cohen, S. Joyce, and J. E. Crowe, Jr. 2016. Cross-neutralizing and protective human antibody specificities to poxvirus infections. *Cell* 167(3):684–694.

Gilead Sciences. I. 2000. *Vistide® (cidofovir injection)*. https://www.accessdata.fda.gov/drugsatfda_docs/label/1999/020638s003lbl.pdf (accessed February 23, 2024).

Grosenbach, D. W., R. Jordan, and D. E. Hruby. 2011. Development of the small-molecule antiviral ST-246 as a smallpox therapeutic. *Future Virology* 6(5):653–671.

Grosenbach, D. W., K. Honeychurch, E. A. Rose, J. Chinsangaram, A. Frimm, B. Maiti, C. Lovejoy, I. Meara, P. Long, and D. E. Hruby. 2018. Oral tecovirimat for the treatment of smallpox. *New England Journal of Medicine* 379(1):44–53.

Gruber, M. F., S. Rubin, and P. R. Krause. 2023. Approaches to demonstrating the effectiveness of filovirus vaccines: Lessons from Ebola and COVID-19. *Frontiers in Immunology* 14:1109486.

Hadfield, J., C. Megill, S. M. Bell, J. Huddleston, B. Potter, C. Callender, P. Sagulenko, T. Bedford, and R. A. Neher. 2018. Nextstrain: Real-time tracking of pathogen evolution. *Bioinformatics* 34(23):4121–4123.

Hammarlund, E., M. W. Lewis, S. V. Carter, I. Amanna, S. G. Hansen, L. I. Strelow, S. W. Wong, P. Yoshihara, J. M. Hanifin, and M. K. Slifka. 2005. Multiple diagnostic techniques identify previously vaccinated individuals with protective immunity against monkeypox. *Nature Medicine* 11(9):1005–1011.

Henderson, D. A., and P. Klepac. 2013. Lessons from the eradication of smallpox: An interview with D. A. Henderson. *Philosophical Transactions of the Royal Society of London, B: Biological Sciences* 368(1623):20130113.

HHS (Department of Health and Human Services). 2023. *Public Health Emergency Medical Countermeasures Enterprise multiyear budget: Fiscal years 2022–2026*. https://aspr.hhs.gov/PHEMCE/Documents/2022-2026-PHEMCE-Budget.pdf (accessed February 18, 2024).

Hou, F., Y. Zhang, X. Liu, Y. M. Murand, J. Xu, Z. Yu, X. Hua, Y. Song, J. Ding, H. Huang, R. Zhao, W. Jia., and X. Yang. 2023. mRNA vaccines encoding fusion proteins of monkeypox virus antigens protect mice from *vaccinia virus* challenge. *Nature Communications* 14(5925).

Hruby, D. 2023. TPOXX: An orthopox antiviral. Presentation at Meeting 3 of the Committee on Current State of Research, Development, and Stockpiling of Smallpox MCMs of the National Academies. December 14. https://www.nationalacademies.org/event/41411_12-2023_meeting-3-of-the-committee-on-the-current-state-of-research-development-and-stockpiling-of-smallpox-medical-countermeasures (accessed February 23, 2024).

Huston, J., S. Curtis, and E. F. Egelund. 2023. Brincidofovir: A novel agent for the treatment of smallpox. *Annals of Pharmacotherapy* 57(10):1198–1206.

Hutchins, S. S., I. Sulemana, K. L. Heilpern, W. Schaffner, G. Wax, E. B. Lerner, B. Watson, R. Baltimore, R. A. Waltenburg, D. Aronsky, S. Coffin, G. Ng, A. S. Craig, A. Behrman, J. Meek, E. Sherman, S. S. Chavez, R. Harpaz, and S. Schmid. 2008. Performance of an algorithm for assessing smallpox risk among patients with rashes that may be confused with smallpox. *Clinical Infectious Disease* 46(Suppl 3):S195–S203.

Hutson, C. L., and I. K. Damon. 2010. Monkeypox virus infections in small animal models for evaluation of anti-poxvirus agents. *Viruses* 2(12):2763–2776.

IOM (Institute of Medicine). 2002. *Scientific and policy considerations in developing smallpox vaccination options: A workshop report*. Washington, DC: The National Academies Press.

IOM. 2005. *The smallpox vaccination program: Public health in an age of terrorism*. Washington, DC: The National Academies Press.

IOM. 2009. *Live variola virus: Considerations for continuing research*. Washington, DC: The National Academies Press.

IOM and NRC (National Research Council). 2011. *BioWatch and public health surveillance: Evaluating systems for the early detection of biological threats: Abbreviated version*. Washington, DC: The National Academies Press.

Jordan, R., J. M. Leeds, S. Tyavanagimatt, and D. E. Hruby. 2010. Development of ST-246® for treatment of poxvirus infections. *Viruses* 2(11):2409–2435.

Kaplan, E. H., D. L. Craft, and L. M. Wein. 2002. Emergency response to a smallpox attack: The case for mass vaccination. *Proceedings of the National Academy of Sciences* 99(16):10935–10940.

Karem, K. L., M. Reynolds, Z. Braden, G. Lou, N. Bernard, J. Patton, and I. K. Damon. 2005. Characterization of acute-phase humoral immunity to monkeypox: Use of immunoglobulin M enzyme-linked immunosorbent assay for detection of monkeypox infection during the 2003 North American outbreak. *Clinical and Diagnostic Laboratory Immunology* 12(7):867–872.

Kausar, S., F. Said Khan, M. Ishaq Mujeeb Ur Rehman, M. Akram, M. Riaz, G. Rasool, A. Hamid Khan, I. Saleem, S. Shamim, and A. Malik. 2021. A review: Mechanism of action of antiviral drugs. *International Journal of Immunopathology and Pharmacology* 35:20587384211002621.

Kennedy, R. B., and P. A. Gregory. 2023. Chapter 55: Smallpox and vaccinia. In W. Orenstein, P. Offit, K. M. Edwards, and S. Plotkin (eds.), *Plotkin's vaccines (8th edition)*. Philadelphia: Elsevier. Pp. 1057–1086.

Khoury, D. S., T. E. Schlub, D. Cromer, M. Steain, Y. Fong, P. B. Gilbert, K. Subbarao, J. A. Triccas, S. J. Kent, and M. P. Davenport. 2023. Correlates of protection, thresholds of protection, and immunobridging among persons with SARS-CoV-2 infection. *Emerging Infectious Diseases* 29(2):381–388.

Ko, K. K. K., K. R. Chng, and N. Nagarajan. 2022. Metagenomics-enabled microbial surveillance. *Nature Microbiology* 7(4):486–496.

Kost, G. J. 2021. Public health education should include point-of-care testing: Lessons learned from the COVID-19 pandemic. *eJIFCC* 32(3):311–327.

Lane, J. M. 2006. Mass vaccination and surveillance/containment in the eradication of smallpox. *Current Topics in Microbiology Immunology* 304:17–29.

Lane, J. M., F. L. Ruben, J. M. Neff, and J. D. Millar. 1969. Complications of smallpox vaccination, 1968: National surveillance in the United States. *New England Journal of Medicine* 281(22):1201–1208.

Lane, J. M., F. L. Ruben, J. M. Neff, and J. Millar. 1970. Complications of smallpox vaccination, 1968: Results of ten statewide surveys. *The Journal of Infectious Diseases* 122(4):303–309.

Lewis, R. 2023. Variola virus research: Overview of main activities and use of live virus. Presentation at Meeting 2 of the Committee on Current State of Research, Development, and Stockpiling of Smallpox MCMs of the National Academies. December 1. https://www.nationalacademies.org/event/41410_12-2023_meeting-2-of-the-committee-on-the-current-state-of-research-development-and-stockpiling-of-smallpox-medical-countermeasures (accessed February 23, 2024).

Li, J., I. Hosegood, D. Powell, B. Tscharke, J. Lawler, K. V. Thomas, and J. F. Mueller. 2023. A global aircraft-based wastewater genomic surveillance network for early warning of future pandemics. *The Lancet Global Health* 11(5):e791–e795.

Li, P., J. A. Al-Tawfiq, Z. A. Memish, and Q. Pan. 2023. Preventing drug resistance: Combination treatment for mpox. *Lancet* 402(10414):1750–1751.

Li, Y., V. A. Olson, T. Laue, M. T. Laker, and I. K. Damon. 2006. Detection of monkeypox virus with real-time PCR assays. *Journal of Clinical Virology* 36(3):194–203.

Li, Z., A. Sinha, Y. Zhang, N. Tanner, H. T. Cheng, P. Premsrirut, and C. K. S. Carlow. 2023. Extraction-free LAMP assays for generic detection of old world orthopoxviruses and specific detection of mpox virus. *Scientific Reports* 13(1):21093.

Lin, D., Y. Shen, and T. Liang. 2023. Oncolytic virotherapy: Basic principles, recent advances and future directions. *Signal Transduction and Targeted Therapy* 8(1):156.

Mack, T. M., J. Nobel, Jr., and D. B. Thomas. 1972. A prospective study of serum antibody and protection against smallpox. *The American Journal of Tropical Medicine and Hygiene* 21(2):214–218.

Martins, K. 2023. Smallpox therapeutics overview. Presentation at Meeting 3 of the Committee on Current State of Research, Development, and Stockpiling of Smallpox MCMs of the National Academies. December 14. https://www.nationalacademies.org/event/41411_12-2023_meeting-3-of-the-committee-on-the-current-state-of-research-development-and-stockpiling-of-smallpox-medical-countermeasures (accessed February 23, 2024).

Mazurkov, O. Y., A. S. Kabanov, L. N. Shishkina, A. A. Sergeev, M. O. Skarnovich, N. I. Bormotov, M. A. Skarnovich, A. S. Ovchinnikova, K. A. Titova, D. O. Galahova, L. E. Bulychev, A. A. Sergeev, O. S. Taranov, B. A. Selivanov, A. Y. Tikhonov, E. L. Zavjalov, A. P. Agafonov, and A. N. Sergeev. 2016. New effective chemically synthesized anti-smallpox compound NIOCH-14. *Journal of General Virology* 97(5):1229–1239.

Merchlinsky, M., A. Albright, V. Olson, H. Schiltz, T. Merkeley, C. Hughes, B. Petersen, and M. Challberg. 2019. The development and approval of tecoviromat (TPOXX®), the first antiviral against smallpox. *Antiviral Research* 168:168–174.

Meyer, H., R. Ehmann, and G. L. Smith. 2020. Smallpox in the post-eradication era. *Viruses* 12(2):138.

Morgan, J., M. H. Roper, L. Sperling, R. A. Schieber, J. D. Heffelfinger, C. G. Casey, J. W. Miller, S. Santibanez, B. Herwaldt, and P. Hightower. 2008. Myocarditis, pericarditis, and dilated cardiomyopathy after smallpox vaccination among civilians in the United States, January–October 2003. *Clinical Infectious Diseases* 46(Suppl3):S242–S250.

Moss, B. 2011. Smallpox vaccines: Targets of protective immunity. *Immunological Reviews* 239(1):8–26.

Mucker, E. M., A. J. Goff, J. D. Shamblin, D. W. Grosenbach, I. K. Damon, J. M. Mehal, R. C. Holman, D. Carroll, N. Gallardo, V. A. Olson, C. J. Clemmons, P. Hudson, and D. E. Hruby. 2013. Efficacy of tecovirimat (ST-246) in nonhuman primates infected with variola virus (smallpox). *Antimicrobial Agents and Chemotherapy* 57(12):6246–6253.

Murphy, J. G., R. S. Wright, G. K. Bruce, L. M. Baddour, M. A. Farrell, W. D. Edwards, H. Kita, and L. T. Cooper. 2003. Eosinophilic–lymphocytic myocarditis after smallpox vaccination. *The Lancet* 362(9393):1378–1380.

Neff, J. M., J. M. Lane, J. H. Pert, R. Moore, J. D. Millar, and D. A. Henderson. 1967a. Complications of smallpox vaccination: National survey in the United States, 1963. *New England Journal of Medicine* 276(3):125–132.

Neff, J. M., R. H. Levine, J. M. Lane, E. A. Ager, H. Moore, B. J. Rosenstein, J. D. Millar, and D. A. Henderson. 1967b. Complications of smallpox vaccination, United States 1963: II. Results obtained by four statewide surveys. *Pediatrics* 39(6):916–923.

NIH (National Institutes of Health). 2022. *Decades in the making: mRNA COVID-19 vaccines.* https://covid19.nih.gov/nih-strategic-response-covid-19/decades-making-mrna-covid-19-vaccines (accessed March 4, 2024).

Oghuan, J., C. Chavarria, S. R. Vanderwal, A. Gitter, A. A. Ojaruega, C. Monserrat, C. X. Bauer, E. L. Brown, S. J. Cregeen, J. Deegan, B. M. Hanson, M. Tisza, H. I. Ocaranza, J. Balliew, A. W. Maresso, J. Rios, E. Boerwinkle, K. D. Mena, and F. Wu. 2023. Wastewater analysis of mpox virus in a city with low prevalence of mpox disease: An environmental surveillance study. *The Lancet Regional Health–Americas* 28:100639.

Olson, V. A., and S. N. Shchelkunov. 2017. Are we prepared in case of a possible smallpox-like disease emergence? *Viruses* 9(9):242. https://doi.org/10.3390/v9090242.

Orlova, O. V., D. V. Glazkova, E. V. Bogoslovskaya, G. A. Shipulin, and S. M. Yudin. 2022. Development of modified vaccinia virus Ankara-based vaccines: Advantages and applications. *Vaccines (Basel)* 10(9):1516.

Overton, E. T., J. Stapleton, I. Frank, S. Hassler, P. A. Goepfert, D. Barker, E. Wagner, A. von Krempelhuber, G. Virgin, T. P. Meyer, J. Müller, N. Bädeker, R. Grünert, P. Young, S. Rösch, J. Maclennan, N. Arndtz-Wiedemann, and P. Chaplin. 2015. Safety and immunogenicity of modified vaccinia Ankara-Bavarian Nordic smallpox vaccine in vaccinia-naive and experienced human immunodeficiency virus-infected individuals: An open-label, controlled clinical phase II trial. *Open Forum Infectious Diseases* 2(2):ofv040.

Parrino, J., L. H. McCurdy, B. D. Larkin, I. J. Gordon, S. E. Rucker, M. E. Enama, R. A. Koup, M. Roederer, R. T. Bailer, Z. Moodie, L. Gu, L. Yan, and B. S. Graham. 2007. Safety, immunogenicity and efficacy of modified vaccinia Ankara (MVA) against Dryvax challenge in vaccinia-naïve and vaccinia-immune individuals. *Vaccine* 25(8):1513–1525.

Peiró-Mestres, A., I. Fuertes, D. Camprubí-Ferrer, M. Marcos, A. Vilella, M. Navarro, L. Rodriguez-Elena, J. Riera, A. Català, M. J. Martínez, and J. L. Blanco. 2022. Frequent detection of monkeypox virus DNA in saliva, semen, and other clinical samples from 12 patients, Barcelona, Spain, May to June 2022. *Euro Surveillance* 27(28):2200503.

Petersen, B. W., I. K. Damon, C. A. Pertowski, D. Meaney-Delman, J. T. Guarnizo, R. H. Beigi, K. M. Edwards, M. C. Fisher, S. E. Frey, R. Lynfield, and R. E. Willoughby. 2015. Clinical guidance for smallpox vaccine use in a postevent vaccination program. *Morbidity and Mortality Weekly Report Recommendations and Reports* 64(2):1–32.

Phetsouphanh, C., D. R. Darley, D. B. Wilson, A. Howe, C. M. L. Munier, S. K. Patel, J. A. Juno, L. M. Burrell, S. J. Kent, G. J. Dore, A. D. Kelleher, and G. V. Matthews. 2022. Immunological dysfunction persists for 8 months following initial mild-to-moderate SARS-CoV-2 infection. *Nature Immunology* 23(2):210–216.

Pinnetti, C., E. Cimini, V. Mazzotta, G. Matusali, A. Vergori, A. Mondi, M. Rueca, S. Batzella, E. Tartaglia, A. Bettini, S. Notari, M. Rubino, M. Tempestilli, C. Pareo, L. Falasca, F. Del Nonno, A. Scarabello, M. Camici, R. Gagliardini, E. Girardi, F. Vaia, F. Maggi, C. Agrati, and A. Antinori. 2023. Mpox as AIDS-defining event with a severe and protracted course: Clinical, immunological, and virological implications. *The Lancet Infectious Diseases* 24(2):e127–e135.

Pittman, P. R., M. Hahn, H. S. Lee, C. Koca, N. Samy, D. Schmidt, J. Hornung, H. Weidenthaler, C. R. Heery, T. P. H. Meyer, G. Silbernagl, J. Maclennan, and P. Chaplin. 2019. Phase 3 efficacy trial of modified vaccinia Ankara as a vaccine against smallpox. *New England Journal of Medicine* 381(20):1897–1908. https://doi.org/10.1056/NEJMoa1817307.

Ratner, L. H., J. M. Lane, and C. N. Vicéns. 1970. Complications of smallpox vaccination: Surveillance during an island-wide program in Puerto Rico, 1967–1968. *American Journal of Epidemiology* 91(3):278–285.

Reeves, P. M., B. Bommarius, S. Lebeis, S. McNulty, J. Christensen, A. Swimm, A. Chahroudi, R. Chavan, M. B. Feinberg, D. Veach, W. Bornmann, M. Sherman, and D. Kalman. 2005. Disabling poxvirus pathogenesis by inhibition of Abl-family tyrosine kinases. *Nature Medicine* 11(7):731–739.

Reeves, P. M., S. K. Smith, V. A. Olson, S. H. Thorne, W. Bornmann, I. K. Damon, and D. Kalman. 2011. Variola and monkeypox viruses utilize conserved mechanisms of virion motility and release that depend on Abl and SRC family tyrosine kinases. *Journal of Virology* 85(1):21–31.

Ristanovic, E., A. Gligic, S. Atanasievska, V. Protic-Djokic, D. Jovanovic, and M. Radunovic. 2016. Smallpox as an actual biothreat: Lessons learned from its outbreak in ex-Yugoslavia in 1972. *Annali dell'Istituto Superiore di Sanita* 52(4):587–597.

Rogers, J. H., K. Newell, B. Westley, and J. Laurence. 2024. Fatal Alaskapox infection in a southcentral Alaska resident. *State of Alaska Epidemiology Bulletin*, February 9. https://epi.alaska.gov/bulletins/docs/b2024_02.pdf (accessed February 22, 2024).

Rosenberg, E. S., V. Dorabawila, R. Hart-Malloy, B. J. Anderson, W. Miranda, T. O'Donnell, C. J. Gonzalez, M. Abrego, C. DelBarba, C. J. Tice, C. McGarry, E. C. Mitchell, M. Boulais, B. Backenson, M. Kharfen, J. McDonald, and U. E. Bauer. 2023. Effectiveness of JYNNEOS vaccine against diagnosed mpox infection—New York, 2022. *Morbidity and Mortality Weekly Report* 72(20):559–563.

Russo, A. T., D. W. Grosenbach, T. L. Brasel, R. O. Baker, A. G. Cawthon, E. Reynolds, T. Bailey, P. J. Kuehl, V. Sugita, K. Agans, and D. E. Hruby. 2018. Effects of treatment delay on efficacy of tecovirimat following lethal aerosol monkeypox virus challenge in cynomolgus macaques. *The Journal of Infectious Diseases* 218(9):1490–1499.

Russo, A. T., A. Berhanu, C. B. Bigger, J. Prigge, P. M. Silvera, D. W. Grosenbach, and D. Hruby. 2020. Co-administration of tecovirimat and ACAM2000™ in non-human primates: Effect of tecovirimat treatment on ACAM2000 immunogenicity and efficacy versus lethal monkeypox virus challenge. *Vaccine* 38(3):644–654.

Ryan, M. A. K., J. F. Seward, and Smallpox Vaccine in Pregnancy Registry Team. 2008. Pregnancy, birth, and infant health outcomes from the national smallpox vaccine in pregnancy registry, 2003–2006. *Clinical Infectious Diseases* 46(Suppl 3):S221–S226.

Sah, R., A. Abdelaal, A. Asija, S. Basnyat, Y. R. Sedhai, S. Ghimire, S. Sah, D. K. Bonilla-Aldana, and A. J. Rodriguez-Morales. 2022. Monkeypox virus containment: The application of ring vaccination and possible challenges. *Journal of Travel Medicine* 29(6):taac085.

Saravanan, K. A., M. Panigrahi, H. Kumar, D. Rajawat, S. S. Nayak, B. Bhushan, and T. Dutt. 2022. Role of genomics in combating COVID-19 pandemic. *Gene* 823:146387.

Sarkar, J. K., A. C. Mitra, M. K. Mukherjee, S. K. De, and D. G. Mazumdar. 1973. Virus excretion in smallpox. 1. Excretion in the throat, urine, and conjunctiva of patients. *Bulletin of the World Health Organization* 48(5):517–522.

Seaman, M. S., M. B. Wilck, L. R. Baden, S. R. Walsh, L. E. Grandpre, C. Devoy, A. Giri, L. C. Noble, J. A. Kleinjan, K. E. Stevenson, H. T. Kim, and R. Dolin. 2010. Effect of vaccination with modified vaccinia Ankara (ACAM3000) on subsequent challenge with Dryvax. *Journal of Infectious Diseases* 201(9):1353–1360.

Sharma, S., J. Pannu, S. Chorlton, J. L. Swett, and D. J. Ecker. 2023. Threat Net: A metagenomic surveillance network for biothreat detection and early warning. *Health Security* 21(5)347–357.

Siegrist, C. M., S. M. Kinahan, T. Settecerri, A. C. Greene, and J. L. Santarpia. 2020. CRISPR/Cas9 as an antiviral against orthopoxviruses using an AAV vector. *Scientific Reports* 10(1)19307.

Siegrist, E. A., and J. Sassine. 2023. Antivirals with activity against mpox: A clinically oriented review. *Clinical Infectious Diseases* 76(1):155–164.

Skiest, D. J., M. Duong, S. Park, L. Wei, and P. Keiser. 1999. Complications of therapy with intravenous cidofovir: Severe nephrotoxicity and anterior uveitis. *Infectious Diseases in Clinical Practice* 8(3):151–157.

Smith, T. G., C. M. Gigante, N. T. Wynn, A. Matheny, W. Davidson, Y. Yang, R. E. Condori, K. O'Connell, L. Kovar, T. L. Williams, Y. C. Yu, B. W. Petersen, N. Baird, D. Lowe, Y. Li, P. S. Satheshkumar, and C. L. Hutson. 2023. Tecovirimat resistance in mpox patients, United States, 2022–2023. *Emerging Infectious Diseases* 29(12):2426–2432.

Suthar, A. B., S. Schubert, J. Garon, A. Couture, A. M. Brown, and S. Charania. 2022. Coronavirus disease case definitions, diagnostic testing criteria, and surveillance in 25 countries with highest reported case counts. *Emerging Infectious Diseases* 28(1):148–156.

Tack, D. M., K. L. Karem, J. R. Montgomery, L. Collins, M. G. Bryant-Genevier, R. Tiernan, M. Cano, P. Lewis, R. J. Engler, I. K. Damon, and M. G. Reynolds. 2013. Unintentional transfer of vaccinia virus associated with smallpox vaccines: ACAM2000® compared with Dryvax®. *Human Vaccines & Immunotherapeutics* 9(7):1489–1496.

Taub, D. D., W. B. Ershler, M. Janowski, A. Artz, M. L. Key, J. McKelvey, D. Muller, B. Moss, L. Ferrucci, P. L. Duffey, and D. L. Longo. 2008. Immunity from smallpox vaccine persists for decades: A longitudinal study. *American Journal of Medicine* 121(12):1058–1064.

Ulaeto, D. O., S. G. Lonsdale, S. M. Laidlaw, G. C. Clark, P. Horby, and M. W. Carroll. 2022. A prototype lateral flow assay for detection of orthopoxviruses. *Lancet Infectious Diseases* 22(9):1279–1280.

WHO (World Health Organization). 2023. Meeting of the Strategic Advisory Group of Experts on Immunization, September 2023: Conclusions and recommendations. *Weekly Epidemiological Record* 47:599–620. https://iris.who.int/bitstream/handle/10665/374327/WER9847-eng-fre.pdf?sequence=1 (accessed February 23, 2024).

WHO. 2024. *154th session of the executive board, provisional agenda item 18—Smallpox eradication: Destruction of variola virus stocks (January 2, 2024).* https://apps.who.int/gb/ebwha/pdf_files/EB154/B154_20-en.pdf (accessed February 23, 2024).

Wolfe, D. 2023. Smallpox vaccines overview. Presentation at Meeting 3 of the Committee on Current State of Research, Development, and Stockpiling of Smallpox MCMs of the National Academies. December 14. https://www.nationalacademies.org/event/41411_12-2023_meeting-3-of-the-committee-on-the-current-state-of-research-development-and-stockpiling-of-smallpox-medical-countermeasures (accessed February 23, 2024).

Yang, G., D. C. Pevear, M. H. Davies, M. S. Collett, T. Bailey, S. Rippen, L. Barone, C. Burns, G. Rhodes, S. Tohan, J. W. Huggins, R. O. Baker, R. L. Buller, E. Touchette, K. Waller, J. Schriewer, J. Neyts, E. DeClercq, K. Jones, D. Hruby, and R. Jordan. 2005. An orally bioavailable antipox-virus compound (ST-246) inhibits extracellular virus formation and protects mice from lethal orthopoxvirus challenge. *Journal of Virology* 79(20):13139–13149.

Zitzmann-Roth, E. M., F. Von Sonnenburg, S. De La Motte, N. Arndtz-Wiedemann, A. Von Krem-pelhuber, N. Uebler, J. Vollmar, G. Virgin, and P. Chaplin. 2015. Cardiac safety of modified vaccinia Ankara for vaccination against smallpox in a young, healthy study population. *PLOS One* 10(4):e0122653.

3

Factors Influencing Smallpox Readiness and Response

"There are two opportunities right now for smallpox medical countermeasures research and development—the opportunity to innovate in manufacturing with a direct impact on what we can stockpile in the future, and the opportunity to better understand the safety and efficacy of these products in the context of mpox response."

Matthew Hepburn, in presentation to the committee
December 15, 2023

Federal smallpox planning in the post-eradication era has been characterized by strategies to reduce the risk that an outbreak would pose, primarily through containment using medical countermeasures (MCMs). Risk reduction can be approached by diminishing the threat itself, the vulnerability to the threat, or the consequences of the threat once it has materialized. The U.S. government has heavily invested in the stockpiling of smallpox vaccine, an MCM risk reduction approach intended to reduce population vulnerability after an outbreak has been detected. The effectiveness of smallpox MCMs (whether diagnostics, vaccines, or therapeutics) as agents of risk reduction rests on numerous factors, from a working knowledge of smallpox biology and epidemiology to the risks and benefits of emerging science and technology to myriad operational planning decisions. Hence, the clinical efficacy of MCMs alone is insufficient to predict its risk-reduction efficacy in an actual outbreak, as MCM distribution and uptake depend on many fiscal, operational, social, and political considerations. These latter considerations, while central, fall outside the scope of this committee, which has focused its efforts on the countermeasures themselves. Similarly, sociopolitical, lab safety, and other strategies to reduce the risk of a small-pox outbreak taking place are also outside the scope. Still, the findings or conclusions related to MCMs in this report should be viewed holistically and as operating within these other considerations.

EVOLVING BIOTHREAT LANDSCAPE

As noted by the World Health Organization (WHO) Advisory Committee on Variola Virus Research (ACVVR) in 2023, the context for smallpox read-iness has changed due to a dramatically different risk landscape, including changes in population (e.g., demographic, physiological, and behavioral/risk perception), since eradication and especially so in recent years:

> Salient elements included the waning of immunity against smallpox in the global population, the advent of the HIV/AIDS pandemic and greater prevalence of other immunosuppressive conditions, the continuing advance of synthetic biology and biotechnology making de novo synthesis of viral pathogens possible, the continuing evolution of orthopoxviruses including genetic features suggesting adaptation to more efficient human-to-human transmission, and the observation that currently available countermeasures may not be sufficient to contain outbreaks in the face of a more transmis-sible and pathogenic orthopoxvirus (WHO, 2024a).

Routine smallpox vaccination ended in 1972 in the United States and globally by 1984. While some studies suggest that protection from vaccination during eradication efforts may be long-lasting, the extent to which this is the case is not well understood, and the durability of vac-cination against clinical smallpox for all current vaccines is unknown (Hammarlund et al., 2003; Taub et al., 2008). While there was a brief attempt to vaccinate a larger fraction of the potentially at-risk civilian population against smallpox in the months leading up to the war in Iraq, this effort largely failed for sociopolitical reasons (IOM, 2005). Presently, only individuals with occupational health risk to smallpox and orthopox-viruses receive inoculation, such as laboratory and health care personnel working with orthopoxviruses and around 1.4 million current and former U.S. military members who could potentially provide essential services in the event of a smallpox outbreak (Decker, et al., 2021; Grabenstein and Winkenwerder, 2003; Petersen et al., 2016). There are questions about duration of protection among non-military U.S. personnel vaccinated since 1972 due to improper application of the scarification technique used for vaccine administration (Kennedy and Gregory, 2023). Individuals who have been vaccinated against mpox using modified vaccinia Ankara-Bavarian Nordic (MVA-BN) are expected to have protection against small-pox (though some scientists posit that the decline of immunity to variola may be a contributing factor in the rising frequency of mpox outbreaks (Durski et al., 2018; Van Dijck et al., 2023)). Therefore, the population of individuals who have been vaccinated with an approved smallpox vaccine since the end of routine vaccination is a very small proportion of the U.S. population. Furthermore, the number of people at risk of serious adverse reaction to replicating smallpox vaccine has grown since eradication (e.g., there are more people now living with HIV and taking immunosuppressant drugs) with one study suggesting that approximately 15 percent of the U.S. population is contraindicated to replicating smallpox vaccine, rising to about 38 percent if their household contacts are included (Carlin et al., 2017; Parrino and Graham, 2006).

It has long been known that accidental or deliberate outbreaks remain possible due to existing and allowed viral collections, and even natural outbreaks are at least theoretically possible if there is viable virus in, for example, thawing permafrost, but recent advances in synthetic biology technology now mean that the variola virus or another microbe that could cause smallpox-like illness could be recreated in a laboratory even if all known collections of variola virus were to be verifiably destroyed (Jaschke et al., 2019; Levrier et al., 2023; Noyce et al., 2018; Reardon, 2014, Thi Nhu Thao et al., 2020; WHO, 2015). Furthermore, since routine smallpox vaccination ended in 1972 in the United States and globally in the ensuing years, population-level immunity has waned. Some scientists posit that the decline of immunity to variola may be a contributing factor in the rising frequency of mpox outbreaks (see Box 3-1) (Durski et al., 2018; Van Dijck et al., 2023).

The changing threat landscape is further evidenced by the increasing frequency and scope of orthopoxvirus outbreaks in recent years (Box 3-1). Mpox outbreaks have occurred sporadically in Central and East Africa (clade I) and West Africa (clade II) since the 1970s (WHO, 2023b). However, an increase in cases, coinciding with improved surveillance, was observed in west and central African countries in the last decade, prior to the 2022 multi-country outbreak (Durski, 2018).

As exemplified by the 2022 and 2023 mpox outbreaks, any orthopoxvirus may become more evolutionarily adapted to humans through alterations in characteristics like transmissibility or virulence. A more comprehensive understanding of basic orthopoxvirus biology, virus–host interactions, and interactions among viral proteins and other molecules could support development of safer and more effective vaccines and therapeutics, as described further in this chapter and in Chapter 4.

Comparative Poxvirology and Implications for MCMs

There are twelve species of poxviruses across four poxvirus genera that are known to infect humans—orthopoxvirus, parapoxvirus, yatapoxvirus,

---

BOX 3-1
Notable Orthopoxvirus Outbreaks (as of February 2024)

Mpox

Clade I monkeypox virus outbreaks occur regularly in Cameroon, Central African Republic, and the Democratic Republic of the Congo and sporadically in others (e.g., Sudan, South Sudan).

In 2003, 71 cases (35 confirmed, 36 suspect and probable cases) of clade II monkeypox virus were reported in six U.S. states (Illinois, Indiana, Kentucky, Missouri, Ohio, and Wisconsin) after contact with infected pet prairie dogs housed near imported small mammals from West Africa (CDC, 2003). This was the first time human mpox was reported outside of Africa.

In 2017, clade II monkeypox virus reemerged in Nigeria after almost four decades of no reported cases (Yinka-Ogunleye et al., 2018).

Since 2022 the clade IIb monkeypox virus has spread globally, affecting many countries without previous mpox cases. Transmission was driven via sexual contact among men who have sex with men.

As of January 28, 2023, 13,357 total mpox cases (714 confirmed cases) and 715 suspected mpox deaths having been reported from 22 out of 26 (85 percent) provinces in the Democratic Republic of Congo (WHO, 2023a). This is the highest number of annual cases ever reported, with new cases in geographic areas that had previously not reported mpox, including Kinshasa, Lualaba, and South Kivu. Clade I monkeypox virus has been confirmed among tested cases.

Alaskapox

The first case of Alaskapox virus infection resulting in hospitalization and death was reported in February 2024 (Hedberg, 2024). Since the first human case was discovered in 2015, six additional cases in humans have been confirmed in the Fairbanks area. The probable animal reservoirs include voles and squirrels. To date, no person-to-person transmission has been documented; domestic animals may play a role in spreading the virus (Alaska Department of Health, 2024).

---

and molluscipoxvirus (Table 3-1). Variola virus is a member of the orthopoxvirus genus within the Poxviridae family. Poxviruses are large and possess a single linear, double-stranded DNA molecule of 130–375 kilobase pairs, depending on the species, which can encode more than 200 proteins (Burrell et al., 2017). Only two viral species of poxviruses are obligate human pathogens: variola virus (orthopoxvirus genus) and molluscum contagiosum (molluscipoxvirus genus). Vaccinia, the prototype poxvirus and basis of modern smallpox vaccines, is also a member of the orthopoxvirus genus and has occasionally caused disease in humans following vaccination. Cowpox virus and orf virus (genus parapoxvirus) primarily affect livestock but may also infect humans. Many other viral species across the poxvirus

TABLE 3-1 Poxviruses That Infect Humans

Genus	Virus	Reservoir Hosts	Other Infected Hosts	Geographic Distribution
Orthopoxvirus	Alaskapox	? Voles and squirrels	?	Alaska
	Cowpox	Bank voles, long-tailed (wood) mice	Cats, rats, cattle, zoo animals	Europe, western Asia
	Monkeypox*	? Unknown—likely rodent	Monkeys, zoo animals, prairie dogs	Western, central Africa, worldwide outbreaks
	Vaccinia	?	Rabbits, cows, river buffaloes	?
	Variola*	Humans	None	Eradicated (formerly worldwide)
Parapoxvirus	Bovine papular stomatitis	Cattle	None	Worldwide
	Orf	Sheep, goats	Ruminants	Worldwide
	Pseudocowpox	Cattle (dairy)	None	Worldwide
	Seal parapoxvirus	Seals	None	Worldwide
Yatapoxvirus	Tanapox virus	?	None	Eastern and central Africa
	Yabapox	? Primates	None	Western Africa
Molluscipoxvirus	Molluscum contagiosum	Humans	None	Worldwide

NOTE: Unknown information is indicated with "?"; viruses capable of respiratory routes of human-to-human transmission are indicated with "*".
SOURCES: Table adapted from Satheshkumar and Damon (2021). Cowpox reservoir hosts from Ninove et al. (2009).

genera affect a wide range of animals, including mammals, fish, birds, and reptiles. These viruses have traditionally been named based on the species of first isolation, and these names may not be reflective of the reservoir species or host range (Moss and Smith, 2021).

As noted in Chapter 1, this report primarily discusses the features of orthopoxviruses and implications for MCMs, due to the greater potential for orthopoxviruses to infect humans. However, the committee recognizes the theoretical potential for spillover of other poxviruses to occur from animal reservoirs and cause disease in humans.

The orthopoxvirus genus comprises many of the mammalian viruses and consists of 13 species, including variola virus—which is unique in its human-restricted host range—and monkeypox virus, a zoonotic infection that has caused outbreaks in humans for many decades in certain areas of the world (McInnes et al., 2023; Satheshkumar and Damon, 2021). Diversity among variola virus strains is also present across the species and could have implications for MCM efficacy.

Orthopoxvirus Pathogenesis in Humans

Variety across the orthopoxvirus genus, the adaptation of variola virus to a single host (i.e., humans), and its exceptional virulence together imply the presence of a complex set of mechanisms of pathogenesis as well as a complex relationship between host and pathogen which is poorly understood. Knowledge of smallpox pathogenesis and immunity is limited since many of the tools and concepts of modern immunology were not available when smallpox was eradicated. Hence, the understanding of smallpox protection is largely based on epidemiologic studies and analysis of immune response to immunization with vaccinia virus. A lack of detailed understanding of host–pathogen interactions within these viruses makes it impossible to predict the zoonotic potential for viruses in the genus.

Orthopoxvirus pathogenesis mechanisms are also generally poorly understood, including for variola major and minor, monkeypox virus clades I and II, and other orthopoxviruses. Although genome sequences across orthopoxviruses are very similar, the diseases that these pathogens cause may manifest quite differently in terms of morbidity, symptomatology, and death rates. For example, hemorrhagic smallpox is the least common but most virulent of the five manifestations of smallpox disease and resulted in nearly 100 percent mortality. Hemorrhagic disease may have manifested because of deficient host protective responses. Pregnant women were also susceptible. Prior vaccination was not protective, and subsequent infected individuals developed the same spectrum of clinical manifestations as those exposed to a person with ordinary smallpox. There are no studies reported in the open-source literature regarding modification of clinical disease in the setting of a large, deliberate aerosol release of variola virus. Nonetheless, virus particles acquired by the aerosol route for respiratory pathogens penetrate the lower respiratory tract and cause severe symptoms, even in immunocompetent persons (Yezli and Otter, 2011). While patients with hemorrhagic smallpox have displayed high levels of circulating virus, they were not considered unusually infectious; however, failure to recognize smallpox among patients with hemorrhagic clinical presentation sometimes led to the spread of hospital-acquired infections (Bray and Buller, 2004).

Variola major was observed more commonly than variola minor and resulted in an average case fatality of 30 percent (range, 20-40 percent) during outbreaks in the 20th century, although there was variability even beyond this range (Breman and Henderson, 2002). For variola minor, mortality ranged from 1 to 2 percent (Berche, 2022). Comparatively, mortality from mpox has ranged from 1 to 10 percent depending on the clade and the study, with clade I resulting in higher fatality rates (Gong et al 2022; Jezek and Fenner, 1988). Active surveillance studies in the 1980s revealed a case fatality rate of 9.8 percent among 338 individuals infected with clade I monkeypox virus in the Democratic Republic of the Congo. All deaths were in unvaccinated children (Jezek and Fenner, 1988). In 2023, WHO reported a case fatality rate of 4.8 percent from suspected clade I disease in the Democratic Republic of the Congo (WHO, 2023a). Clade IIa monkeypox virus caused confirmed infections in 37 individuals in the United States in 2003. No mortality was reported (Reynolds et al., 2007). A narrative review of studies regarding the global outbreak of clade IIb monkeypox virus, largely affecting men who report having sex with men, reported a case fatality rate of 0.1 percent (Antinori et al., 2023). Other orthopoxviruses and poxviruses that infect humans, such as cowpox, vaccinia, orf, or molluscum, cause localized disease and minimal morbidity or mortality in immunocompetent people.

Understanding Immune Evasion and Species Tropism

Understanding immune evasion and species tropism allows for a better understanding of viral pathogenesis and might lead to the development of additional therapeutic options. Knowledge of the features of human tropism of variola virus might also produce insights into the potential for "natural" (or unnatural) evolution of a variola-like virus, presenting challenges and opportunities related to dual use research of concern. Understanding host tropism may also aid in the identification of the animal reservoirs of poxviruses, with implication for One Health management approaches.

While poxviruses can bind to and enter a wide range of mammalian cells, their success in replicating depends on a variety of host-related factors, including cell type, cell cycle status, and intracellular signaling events associated with immunity and cellular apoptosis (IOM, 2009b). The study of viral genes that influence host range and the elucidation of their interactions with host proteins and signaling pathways have improved the understanding of tropism. Poxviruses encode many genes that modulate host antiviral responses (Moss and Smith, 2021). These include secreted viral proteins that bind host cytokines, chemokines, and complement proteins as well as intracellular antagonists that block key signaling pathways, thus precluding establishment of an antiviral state, apoptosis, or proinflammatory response (IOM, 2009b). This wide-ranging capacity to antagonize immune responses is likely to be a factor in the exceptional virulence of variola.

A strong affinity for one host species, sometimes referred to as species "tropism," appears to be generally driven by virus genus- and species-specific genes, as opposed to genes in highly conserved regions of the orthopoxvirus genome (Moss and Smith, 2021). Fully one-third to one-half of poxvirus genes are in the immunoregulation/host interaction category, about which we have only limited understanding (Gubser et al., 2004; Smith et al., 2013). Some exciting advances in recent years have improved the understanding to an extent, such as research on myxoma virus in rabbits exploring the virus' interaction with host antiviral protein kinase R (Peng et al., 2016) and with SAMD9, which binds the C7L family of proteins that is widely distributed among poxviruses (Liu et al., 2011). An investigation into SAMD9 showed that it is an anticodon nuclease that inhibits codon-specific protein synthesis (Zhang et al., 2023).

Structure and Replication

Orthopoxviruses possess a characteristic brick-shaped form with internal structures resembling a dumbbell with two lateral bodies. This structure is highly conserved among poxviruses, and its distinctiveness allows for the use of electron microscopy (EM) as a diagnostic tool that reveals the presence of a poxvirus. EM use is limited, however, in that it cannot discriminate between poxviruses (except parapoxviruses when using negative-stain EM) (Petersen and Damon, 2015).

EM has nevertheless revealed a wealth of information about viral structure. Virions are individual viral particles produced through the act of viral replication (Moss and Smith, 2021), and virion structure has important implications for antiviral development, especially as it relates to the mechanisms of cell entry, the knowledge of which has largely been informed through studies of vaccinia.

A unique feature of poxviruses is that they replicate solely in the cytoplasm of infected cells, in cytoplasmic "viral factories" where immature virions are produced. These develop into mature virions (MVs) that are fully infectious and which may be released with cell lysis or may become wrapped by trans-Golgi and endosomal cisternae, then transported to the cell periphery where they can fuse with the plasma membrane and become released as infectious enveloped virions (EVs). These EVs then become infectious to other cells, entering these cells by endocytosis or by fusion at the plasma membrane. Once inside a new cell, the virions act quickly and early mRNA synthesis in the cytoplasm can be detected within 20 minutes as the cycle begins anew (Moss and Smith, 2021). Early mRNAs encode many immunoregulatory proteins, intermediate transcription factors, and DNA replication enzymes/factors. This fast action can help facilitate the rapid spread of virus from cell to cell.

Progression through this life cycle involves the action of a significant number of virally encoded products and the participation of host proteins and intracellular structures. The viral proteins that mediate the lifecycle progression represent potential targets for antiviral therapy (Figure 3-1). Viral proteins may play an important role in viral resistance to therapeutics, such as tecovirimat (Chapter 2), which targets a protein that is vital for MV envelopment into EV and required for cell-to-cell spreading. Antiviral agents developed to date work by interrupting viral DNA replication (cidofovir and brincidofovir) or the envelopment process (tecovirimat). Additional antivirals with distinct mechanisms of action—e.g., directly targeting the virion components and many other steps of viral replication within the host—have not yet been explored for smallpox. The intentional development of such antivirals would benefit from high-resolution images of structures and improved knowledge of virion function and poxvirology. Virion structures and compositions, their immunogenicity, and their mechanisms of function are also critical pieces of information for the support of subunit vaccine development.

As described above, viral replication occurs in the cytoplasm (Moss and Smith, 2021). A process called uncoating aids in the release of DNA from the

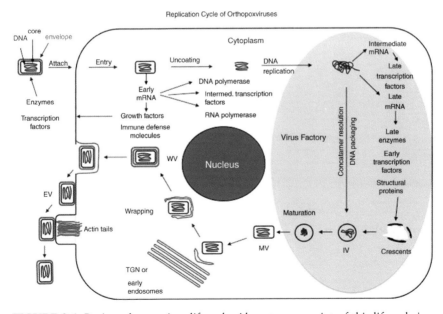

FIGURE 3-1 Basic orthopoxvirus lifecycle. Almost every point of this lifecycle is a potential antiviral target.
SOURCE: Moss and Smith (2021), Figure 16.6. Reproduced with permission.

virus core—DNA that can then serve as the template for DNA replication. The host's proteasome inhibitors can prevent uncoating, a mechanism that is not well understood. The newly synthesized viral DNA serves as the template to transcribe intermediate mRNAs, which encode late transcription factors to initiate late transcription. Intermediate and late mRNAs encode structural proteins. These structural proteins and DNA genomes are assembled into viral particles in a complex process that is not well understood (Moss and Smith, 2021).

Each of these replication steps could be targeted for specific antiviral development, but the understanding of many of these steps is limited. For instance, science has not identified the receptors used for poxvirus entry, and it is possible that poxviruses use an unconventional entry mechanism. In addition, there are many outstanding questions regarding DNA replication, transcription, virion assembly, envelope morphogenesis, and egress. These knowledge gaps present barriers to the further development of specific and novel antivirals, to the improvement of vaccines, and to reducing complications associated with vaccines and therapies.

Orthopoxvirus Evolution and Implications for MCM Utility

Orthopoxvirus evolution appears to have been influenced over time by gene loss, fragmentation, and duplication, with subsequent impacts on such features as virus host range and virulence (IOM, 2009b). One analysis identified 49 conserved genes across 21 members of the Poxviridae family, many of which encode key functions such as replication, transcription, virion assembly, or maturation (Upton et al., 2003). These genes are located toward the central region of the genome, in contrast with the more terminal location of genes that are more virus- or host-interaction-specific.

More recent studies during the 2022 mpox outbreak demonstrated previously unappreciated host–viral characteristics, such as viral gene mutations possibly driven by the host antiviral enzyme APOBEC3, which reveal mechanisms of viral adaptation as well as important clues to the evolution of transmissibility (Ndodo et al., 2023; O'Toole et al., 2023). APOBEC3 may mutate DNA through the short-inverted repeats (IRs) in the viral genome, with one study showing that IRs (not the inverted terminal repeats) are indeed a hot spot for mutation (Dobrovolná et al., 2023).

Within genera of poxviruses, the identification of conserved targets or antigenic epitopes among different poxviruses could facilitate the development of broad-spectrum antivirals and vaccines. It may also be possible to look for more broadly cross-reactive poxvirus targets of drugs and vaccines. Genomic similarity and variation among poxviruses, as well as mutation/deletion/addition, will affect the specificity and sensitivity of PCR-based diagnostic assays.

Utility of Orthopoxviruses for Vaccines and Therapeutics

Importantly, some orthopoxviruses have been used as tools against smallpox. Vaccinia virus, an orthopoxvirus that is the basis of currently licensed smallpox vaccines, was cultivated in laboratories over decades for the purposes of vaccinating against smallpox, though the ancestral orthopoxvirus that it originated from is unknown. Vaccinia virus provides benefits to fight against smallpox and other highly pathogenic orthopoxviruses (Jacobs et al., 2009; Torres-Domínguez and McFadden, 2019). Orthopoxviruses have also been studied for their utility as vaccine and oncolytic virotherapeutic agents against various infectious human and animal diseases and cancers (Pastoret and Vanderplasschen, 2003; Perdiguero et al., 2023).

Remaining Gaps

WHO eradication effort was a remarkable success at eliminating smallpox disease from the human population. Though viral collections remain, the public health feat of the disease's eradication remains an amazing human achievement. The success of that achievement was predicated on the human–host specificity of variola: human-to-human transmission could be successfully interrupted permanently because there was no concern of spillover from another host species and no human chronically infected state.

Yet, considerable gaps remain in understanding variola virus to inform improved MCM development as well as in current understanding of other orthopoxviruses with one or more mammalian reservoir hosts that can infect humans (Moss and Smith, 2021). If speculation that the smallpox virus at one point jumped from animals to human and eventually adapted to be a human-specific pathogen is correct, then other zoonotic poxviruses might follow a similar path of modification to their host tropisms. This represents one possible pathway to renewed outbreaks of smallpox or smallpox-like illness among humans.

Attracting funding for experimental work with smallpox virus to advance more fundamental understandings is challenged by the difficulty of linking such work directly to an "essential" public health need as well as by sociopolitical and ethical concerns about funding dual use research (Damon et al., 2014). The WHO ACVVR has taken a conservative approach to interpreting the World Health Assembly's resolution on approval of research with variola, leading it to use a relatively restrictive lens when deciding whether to approve work with live virus based on what it perceives constitutes an essential public health need. In particular, "discovery research" with live variola virus (VARV) (i.e., research for its own sake), while potentially interesting and useful, is not consistent with the National Academies'

2009 conclusions, which still suggested that targeted basic science research on variola could support better understanding of pathogenesis and human immune response, with direct implications for improved readiness for smallpox and other orthopoxviruses (IOM, 2009b). The disease ecology of the orthopoxviruses is poorly understood. Susceptible species are not infrequently recognized (see Table 3-1). The impact of where infectious exposure occurs likely impacts disease acquisition and transmission. For example, captive zoo animals and prairie dogs have been shown to be susceptible to mpox infection (Jezek and Fenner, 1988). Prairie dogs efficiently transmitted mpox disease to humans in the United States in 2003 (Reynolds et al., 2007). Zoo animals have also been susceptible to cowpox virus infections (Costa et al., 2023). Box 3-2 reveals a suite of poxvirus knowledge gaps that may be relevant for smallpox MCM research, and which is discussed in further detail in Chapter 4 and specifically Table 4-2.

Conclusions on Contribution of Basic Poxvirus Research to Smallpox Readiness

(3-1) The increasing recognition of orthopoxvirus illnesses in humans merits ongoing research and development of MCMs to detect, prevent, treat, and respond to these diseases. This is of particular importance for mpox that is an ongoing global outbreak and is expected to be a long-term threat. Other emerging orthopoxviruses (e.g., Alaskapox, cowpox, and vaccinia-like viruses) also need to be closely monitored as the population immunity against orthopoxviruses continues to wane.

(3-2) Variola virus-specific research is extremely restricted and is only undertaken when it is necessary and essential for public health. It is not possible to fill knowledge gaps without the study of other orthopoxviruses.

(3-3) Gaps exist in the fundamental understanding of variola virus and non-variola orthopoxvirus biology, pathogenesis, immunity and host interactions, evolution, transmission, and ecology. Basic poxvirus research is beneficial to smallpox MCM development and contributes to readiness against other known and potential novel orthopoxviruses affecting humans. General advances in developing orthopoxviruses as vaccine vectors, gene delivery, and oncolytic virotherapy can have multiple benefits, including enhancing smallpox MCMs.

EVOLVING RESEARCH AND TECHNOLOGY LANDSCAPE

As biotechnologies continue to evolve at a remarkable pace—a pace increasingly accelerated by advancements in artificial intelligence—it is incumbent on decision makers to consider what impacts and opportunities may arise for MCM strategies. Malicious exploitation of such technologies

---

BOX 3-2
Poxvirus Knowledge Gaps

Genomics
- Detailed knowledge of genomic evolution.
- Mechanisms for genomic DNA editing that lead to quick adaptation in new hosts.
- Adaptation trends in pathogenesis at the genomic level and tools to forecast future outcomes.

Viral Structure and Replication
- Many aspects of viral lifecycles, e.g., receptor(s) and entry mechanisms, DNA replication mechanism, virion assembly, and egress.
- High-resolution imagery of virion structures and structures at various stages of viral replication.

Immune Responses
- Immunological elements that are central to elevating immunity against new infection.
- Immunodominant antigens/epitopes of all human-infectable poxviruses.
- Host and viral elements that determine breakthrough infections.
- Immunoregulation mechanisms of numerous poxvirus immune evasion proteins.

Host–Pathogen Interactions and Mechanism of Host Tropism
- Knowledge of the hundreds of proteins and their functional interactions with viral and host functions that can shape viral transmission, host range, host immunity, virulence, and pathogenicity.
- Better characterization of factors that determine host range and virulence in cell culture and experimental animal infections.
- Poxvirus species leaping is still in its infancy. Natural reservoirs and the risk of establishment of new reservoirs in novel animal hosts during widespread outbreaks.
- Comprehensive understanding of cellular mechanisms promoting or inhibiting poxvirus adaptation for zoonotic infection and "species leaping."

Other
- Identification of unknown poxviruses.
- Which poxviruses may pose the biggest risk to humans.
- Variants of oncolytic poxviruses that can tumor-target after intravenous delivery.

SOURCES: Personal communication, G. McFadden, Arizona State University *retired*, January 18, 2024; personal communication, Y. Xiang, UT Health San Antonio, January 21, 2024; personal communication, S. Rothenburg, University of California, Davis, January 24, 2024; personal communication, B. Moss, National Institute of Allergy and Infectious Diseases, January 18, 2024; personal communication, J. Liu, University of Arkansas for Medical Sciences, January 26, 2024.

could create novel bioterror agents that render an established MCM ineffective. Beneficial uses, if strategically developed and promulgated, could
significantly mitigate infectious diseases as threats to personal, public, political, and environmental health.

Some argue that the continued existence of live VARV poses obvious
inherent risks, including accidental release, laboratory-acquired infections,
and the deliberate misuse of the virus as a bioterrorism weapon. Efforts to
mitigate these risks involve stringent biosafety and biosecurity measures,
strict multilateral global regulation and oversight of all research with live
virus, and collaboration and transparent communication with the public
and the international community. The exact extent of the risk entailed by
keeping live virus and the effectiveness of various efforts to mitigate these
risks are challenging to assess, while the potential benefits of research using
live virus at the current time are easier to quantify.

Potential Risks of Technological Advancements on MCM Readiness

Synthetic Biology and Gene Editing

Advancements in the fields of synthetic biology and reverse genomics
have shown that infectious viruses (e.g., horsepox virus and SARS-CoV-2)
can be constructed in advanced laboratory settings based on published
genomes (Jaschke et al., 2019; Levrier et al., 2023; Noyce et al., 2018; Thi
Nhu Thao et al., 2020). This suggests that infectious variola virus, or a virus
resembling variola virus, could similarly be re-constructed (Impelluso and
Lentzos, 2017). Modern risk-reduction strategies must therefore account
for the additional risk posed by synthetic biology and gene editing, such as
by ensuring that biosecurity regulations for research with gene sequences of
VARV keep pace with the increasingly available and lower-cost technology
that can be used to produce such sequences (WHO, 2015).

Member companies of the International Gene Synthesis Consortium
have voluntarily committed to screening DNA synthesis orders for sequences aligned with dangerous pathogens, such as those on the U.S. Select
Agent and Toxin List[1] and the Australia Group Common Control List
(Hoffmann et al., 2023). The United States has historically not required
such screening for orders, but could, and the Department of Health and
Human Services (HHS) issued guidance in 2010 recommending baseline
standards for the gene synthesis industry to ensure compliance with Select
Agent Regulations, Export Administration Regulations, and, in general,

---

[1] Federal Select Agent List, https://www.selectagents.gov/sat/list.htm (accessed February 5,
2024).

best practices for addressing biosecurity concerns (HHS, 2010). In February 2024, the International Biosecurity and Biosafety Initiative for Science was launched and intends to collaborate with governments, nongovernmental organizations, industry, and academia to develop shared practices and tools for international bioscience and biotechnology (e.g., cost-effective screening software for DNA synthesis providers) (NTI, 2024). The Biden administration has issued an executive order tasking the Office of Science and Technology Policy to issue a framework to *encourage* providers to implement comprehensive screening mechanisms—but it also *requires* all federal agencies that fund life science research to establish conditions of funding related to synthetic nucleic acid procurement through providers that adhere to the framework (White House, 2023). Stronger legal regulation of gene synthesis could be possible and might appear desirable if access to gene synthesis tools becomes widely availability outside of government-funded labs. The real-world effectiveness of stronger DNA synthesis regulations on preventing mal-intentioned actors from acquiring smallpox or other pathogens by synthesis is unknown and has been called into question (Carlson, 2015).

Regardless, smallpox is unique among pathogens when it comes to the governance of gene synthesis in the United States because possession or work with the virus itself is already subject to stringent regulations. In 2004—when concern over smallpox and other agents that could be used as bioweapons was heightened—Congress passed a terrorism prevention law, signed by President Bush. Title 18, Section 175c of the U.S. criminal code has stated ever since that it is "unlawful for any person to knowingly produce, engineer, synthesize, acquire, transfer directly or indirectly, receive, possess, import, export, or use, or possess and threaten to use, variola virus" (with an exception for work conducted "by, or under the authority of" the HHS secretary).[2] The law goes on to define variola virus as the virus itself or any derivative that contains more than 85 percent of the gene sequence of the variola major or variola minor virus. Variola is the only pathogen that has such an entry in the code. Thus, law enforcement in the United States is already empowered to deter, investigate, and intervene on research or work involving smallpox—and there have been no reported violations of this law in the United States.

While construction of orthopoxvirus from scratch is now possible, the committee estimated that the number of labs capable of carrying out such work is limited to perhaps less than 100 globally. The committee expects this number to increase over the next two decades as DNA synthesis and genome construction techniques improve dramatically. Moreover, the modification of an existing orthopoxvirus to increase virulence has long been possible (Tucker, 2002). Thus, there is an urgent window of opportunity

---

[2] *18 U.S. Code § 175c—Variola virus* (2004).

open now to use both policy and regulatory levers and emerging biotechnologies in developing and deploying next-generation solutions (below) for securing against any potential threats due to increasingly widespread access to synthetic biology capabilities.

Artificial Intelligence

While artificial intelligence (AI) and large language models (LLMs) hold the promise of significant human benefit, these technologies might also pose potential risks to biosecurity and could increase the likelihood of unsanctioned research to re-create smallpox or a virus resembling smallpox (Kuiken, 2023; White House, 2023). While efforts are underway to ensure that LLMs cannot be used to create explicit instructions for planning and executing a biological attack, LLMs could provide assistance in planning the technical details of an attack or by identifying the knowledge to re-create a virus in a laboratory setting (i.e., "AI assistants") (Mouton et al., 2023; Sandbrink, 2023). Another class of AI tools dubbed "biological design tools" also pose potential risk as these tools are trained on biological data and have the capability to create proteins, gene clusters, orgenomes, and it is likely they will have the capability to create more complex biological structures with time (Sandbrink, 2023).

It is not yet clear exactly how such tools may be used or the exact nature of the risks and opportunities resulting. For example, a "long-context language model for the generation of bacteriophage genomes" recently reported development of software that automatically generates bacteriophage-like genomes starting from natural genome sequences (Shao, 2024). Whether any of the so-computed "genomes" encode viable phage is unclear. The committee conducted an ad hoc independent bioinformatic examination of the resulting sequences, which appear to encode phage-like genomes (e.g., open reading frame patterns), but at least some of the resulting open reading frames have no homology to any known proteins. As a second example, Nguyen et al. (2024) reported a 7 billion parameter model with a context length of 131 kilobases capable of generating coding rich sequences over 500 kilobases. De novo generation of Cas-like, transposon-like, and genome-like sequences were reported although, as with Shao, no experimental tests of function were reported. The tool, Evo, also supported mutational and gene essentiality analysis. Taken together, foreseeable advances could increase the likelihood that an AI-based tool could help researchers create viable phage and perhaps other viruses, including pox viruses. Already these tools could also aid researchers in analyzing and understanding pox viruses, natural or otherwise.

However, the impacts of AI-based tools on pox virus research and planning may be limited by the number of available poxvirus genome sequences. There are orders of magnitude more phage and bacteria genome sequences available for training AI models, suggesting potential policy opportunities regarding the sequencing and publishing of any additional poxvirus genome sequences. The convergence of AI, synthetic biology, and reverse genomics might eventually lead to a future where previously unimaginable orthopox viruses could be prototyped in an advanced laboratory setting. These same tools, if well developed and organized in advance, could make understanding and responding to any such virus much easier. Such possibilities seem likely to become more material throughout the 2020s, emphasizing that now is the time to develop robust, resilient, and agile approaches for protecting against malicious or inadvertent future smallpox outbreaks.

Genome Sequencing

Advances in genomic sequencing and computational molecular biology have afforded an improved understanding of the genetic relatedness and evolutionary history of orthopox viruses, though gaps remain. The complete genome sequence of a virulent smallpox strain was first published in 1994 (Massung et al., 1994). Since then, gene sequencing technology has become portable, more accessible, and connected to computing and internet systems facilitating access to this information. Entire genomes can be sequenced in hours instead of weeks. Next-generation sequencing, which is a high-throughput process that allows for the sequencing of genes or genomes in a short timeframe, has enormous potential for its applications for research and diagnostics (Qin, 2019). As of early 2024 the Centers for Disease Control and Prevention (CDC) in the United States and the State Research Center of Virology and Biotechnology (VECTOR) in the Russian Federation have reported complete genome sequencing for, respectively, 40 and 50 smallpox isolates from their collections (WHO, 2023c). At the January 2024 meeting of the WHO executive board the representative of the Russian Federation called attention to potential concerns about making such sequences publicly available (WHO Executive Board, 2024). Thus, like many other technologies, genomic sequencing tools carry dual use potential (i.e., the benefits of learning about genomic variability across smallpox isolates come with the potential harm that sequencing these isolates is a first step toward creating them de novo using the tools below) (NASEM, 2017).

Potential Benefits of Technological Advancements on MCM Readiness

Many innovations in next-generation approaches to infectious disease diagnostics, vaccinations, and treatments, which might have utility in responding to a smallpox outbreak, have been developed around other pathogens. It is important for such innovations to be evaluated and adopted, as useful, for mitigating risks associated with smallpox. As discussed in Chapter 2, isothermal amplification technologies were improved on during the COVID-19 pandemic and 2022 mpox outbreak as a more cost efficient, though less specific, alternative to quantitative polymerase chain reaction (qPCR) (Kaminski et al., 2021). Clustered regularly interspaced short palindromic repeats (CRISPR)-based diagnostics have also been developed to potentially address the need for diagnostic technologies that are cost efficient and maintain diagnostic accuracy (Kaminski et al., 2021). The potential for decentralized biomanufacturing vaccines can be further advanced via the use of lyophilized cell-free extracts (Warfel et al., 2023). More recent developments also suggest that naturally competent microbes can be bioengineered to serve as living sentinels to record the presence of tumors and viral species with health implications in both the environment and people (Cooper et al., 2023; Nou and Voigt, 2024).

Whole-cell synthetic biology has resulted in breakthrough approaches to metabolic engineering, including yeast-based production of complex natural medicinal products (e.g., scopolamine, hyoscyamine) (Srinivasan and Smolke, 2020). As a result, such active pharmaceutical ingredients and biosynthetic key starting materials can be quickly manufactured at scale, without depending on complex synthetic chemistry or agriculture-based supply chains (Antheia, 2024). This suggests that it may be strategically possible to develop future smallpox treatments that can be biosynthesized.

While many questions regarding synthetic mRNA vaccines should be explored (e.g., why immunity is short lived for COVID), next-generation approaches to vaccination continue to be developed. For example, commensal skin microbes have recently been modified to present antigens to the immune system, resulting in initial protection against melanoma in mice (Chen et al., 2023). If such approaches could be developed for smallpox, then vaccine manufacturing and readiness would become much easier to manage.

Taken together, emerging biotechnologies promise rapid, reliable, and local production of diagnostics, treatments, and vaccines. If this comes to pass, then future readiness could be less oriented around maintaining massive physical stockpiles of finished products and more focused on developing and proving the capacities to respond and deploy on demand, when and where needed (Hepburn, 2023). Realizing this future would require significant strategic leadership, coordination, and investment.

The COVID-19 pandemic and the mpox outbreak spurred significant research and development efforts for vaccines, biologics, therapeutics, and diagnostic tools. Lessons learned from these experiences can inform the evaluation of smallpox MCMs and illustrate the potential value of investing in innovative technologies.

A non-exhaustive list of additional tools that could help develop a more forward-looking approach to smallpox readiness includes:

- *Artificial intelligence*: for instance, protein structure prediction (alpha-fold) and bioinformatics. These AI technologies have enabled such advances as protein structure modeling used to understand proteins' function and evolutional histories and to identify potential drug targets (Mutz et al., 2023).
- *Genome sequencing*: rapid growth in next-generation sequencing has made possible the rapid identification of pathogens, the monitoring of drug-resistance mutations and dominant strains/variants, and the suggestion of evolutionary mechanisms and directions, and has facilitated the epidemiologic tracking of transmission (GAO, 2021; Grad and Lipsitch, 2014; Jauneikaite et al., 2023).
- *Proteomics*: the study of the entire complement of proteins expressed by a virus has provided more in-depth understanding of viral structure and biology and may provide novel targets or strategies for MCMs (Zubair et al., 2022).
- *Lipidomic profiling*: similar to proteomics, lipidomics has elucidated the lipid profiles required for viral replication, which may suggest novel antiviral targets (Martín-Acebes et al., 2019; Yuan et al., 2019).
- *Super-resolution microscopy and imaging*: tools like cryogenic electron microscopy, cryo-electron tomography, and super-resolution imaging have the potential to identify antiviral targets with novel mechanisms of action.
- *CRISPR*: CRISPR-based antivirals could offer broad-spectrum therapeutics for all orthopoxvirus species (Mayes, 2023). CRISPR technology has also been applied to mpox diagnostics (Jiang et al., 2023).

Conclusions on Benefits and Risks of Scientific and Technological Advances

(3-4) The potential exists to synthesize the complete or partial variola virus genome and to manufacture infectious viral particles based on published genomes. Targeted modifications to the genome are also possible, which could alter functional components of the virus that could affect transmissibility or virulence. This capacity means that even the guaranteed complete eradication of all existing smallpox collections today would not guarantee against its re-emergence as a threat. It also introduces greater challenges in readiness planning by introducing the possibility of atypical epidemiological or clinical presentations of the disease.

(3-5) Advances in emerging biotechnologies could also allow for the rapid development and deployment of MCMs. A global, real-time, distributed, manufacturing network could enable safe and equitable production of smallpox diagnostics, vaccines, and therapeutics when and where needed to rapidly bring an outbreak anywhere in the world under control. A strategic research and development program promoting the development of general capability in this regard has the potential to unlock such a future.

OPERATIONAL CONSIDERATIONS FOR MCM READINESS AND RESPONSE

The U.S. MCM enterprise is a complex system that includes public and private entities that develop, manufacture, store, distribute, and administer MCMs. COVID-19 and mpox underscored the importance of an effectively coordinated MCM enterprise and highlighted significant gaps in federal readiness (NASEM, 2021). And while the smallpox portfolio is relatively mature compared to other products in the U.S. Strategic National Stockpile (SNS), these products have never been deployed in response to an actual smallpox outbreak so it is unknown how well the system will perform, to what extent smallpox MCMs will reach intended end users, and how front-line responders and laboratories will manage the influx of smallpox cases.

Manufacturing Capacity

While modern manufacturing of smallpox MCMs has advanced significantly since the "animal vaccine" farms of the late 19th century (Esparza et al., 2020), the SNS still relies on just a few manufacturers, so the failure of just one entity to deliver needed MCMs could undermine readiness and response. If the SNS administrators were to undertake an assessment of the proportion of the SNS's smallpox MCM holdings produced by each company and how the loss of manufacturing capacity from any given company could affect readiness for full-scale population needs, it could inform decisions about whether investment from the Biomedical Advanced Research and Development Authority and SNS should be further diversified across more companies and other strategies to the ensure stability of the manufacturing base. One concerning situation could be the potential for a country to prohibit any export of MCM required to respond to a smallpox outbreak. To mitigate this scenario, the Administration for Strategic Preparedness and Response (ASPR) could consider options that would allow onshore manufacturing of products that normally originate outside the United States in such conditions. For example, a manufacturer could be required under contract to establish a relationship with a U.S.-based, large molecule contract development and manufacturing organization (CDMO) to produce additional product on their behalf in a global crisis.

For all smallpox MCMs, questions remain on whether there is sufficient capacity to scale MCM production in the event of a large-scale smallpox event, considering decades of supply chain disruption and shortages as well as the time-intensive regulatory processes that ensure safety and efficacy of medical products (NASEM, 2022a,b). For example, lengthy lead times to obtain raw materials are a critical issue for scaling manufacturing capacity. Emergent BioSolutions reported that if the company did not continually maintain raw materials, component parts, and existing staff, it could take upward of 2 years for additional ACAM2000 vaccines to become available following a procurement request (Sinclair, 2023). Further, while the actual manufacturing of vaccine may only take days, release testing can take up to 9 months to satisfy U.S. Food and Drug Administration (FDA) requirements (Chaplin, 2023).

The COVID-19 pandemic offers salient lessons for countermeasure availability. Once the pandemic began, the mechanism the U.S. government used was Operation Warp Speed (OWS). Enabled by a June 2020 memorandum of understanding between HHS and the Department of Defense (DoD), OWS was a joint effort to accelerate the development, production, and distribution of COVID-19 vaccines, which involved hundreds of staff from across the two departments (GAO, 2022). In January 2022, the Government Accountability Office (GAO) identified lessons learned from OWS. Among the positive decisions made by OWS, GAO cited investment diversification across multiple companies using different platform technologies and parallel investment in large-scale manufacturing while clinical trials were still ongoing (GAO, 2022).

Some options to ensure commercial manufacturing capability might include support for warm-base and just-in-time manufacturing (NASEM, 2016). Steps such as these can help foster vaccine availability at points of need during the initial period of identification of a smallpox outbreak. The commercialization of cross-protective orthopoxvirus MCMs would also be an important step: It would be attractive to industry, would inherently provide a warm base from which to support an emergency manufacturing response, and would ground a system of establishment and replenishment of vendor-managed inventory of cached vaccine (or raw vaccine material). The expected 2024 commercialization of MVA-BN for the purpose of controlling mpox in the United States, for instance, may enable greater availability of the vaccine for a smallpox emergency. Advances in the use of poxviruses as vaccine vectors, for gene delivery, and as oncolytic virotherapy might also bring benefits for enhancing smallpox MCMs, and these might also attract commercial resources and therefore enhance the smallpox response capability.

In 2012, HHS established the Centers for Innovation in Advanced Development and Manufacturing (CIADM), composed of three physical manufacturing sites, to improve domestic infrastructure and expertise to produce MCMs in response to public health emergencies. Among other challenges, the program lacked sustained funding and regular manufacturing work to prepare for a real-world response and, during the COVID-19 pandemic, faced challenges with reliably producing products at scale (GAO, 2023). HHS has ended the CIADM program and is transitioning to a new national Biopharmaceutical Manufacturing Preparedness Consortium (Bio-MaP), a consortium-based approach of industry partners working together with government through flexible contracting authorities to expand the industrial and manufacturing base. It is not entirely clear how HHS will avoid some of the same challenges that faced CIADM, and the new model will require appropriate and sustained funding, rapid federal agency contracting capacity, and relevant expertise. In 2020, DoD granted the BioIndustrial Manufacturing and Design Ecosystem (BioMADE) an award for a new Manufacturing Innovation Institute to collaborate with public and private entities and advance sustainable manufacturing capabilities for the U.S. bioindustrial base (DoD, 2020).

Access and Uptake

The successes of OWS in developing safe and effective vaccines for COVID-19 in record time were tempered by major issues with accessibility and uptake domestically and globally. The billions of U.S. dollars invested in research and development for COVID-19 vaccines helped turn the tide against serious illness and hospitalization, while also revealing a level of vaccine hesitancy and differential uptake across the United States that had not been planned for (CDC, 2023; Kates et al., 2022; Robinson et al., 2022). In addition to hesitancy, uptake was also influenced by access. A 2022 Kaiser Family Foundation (KFF) analysis of Paxlovid and another oral therapy being used under an Emergency Use Authorization, Lagevrio (molnupiravir), found disparities in access to at-home orally administered treatments in the United States, with impoverished counties and individuals who were majority Black, Hispanic, or American Indian or Alaska Native facing reduced access—the same populations that disproportionately suffered poor COVID-19 outcomes (Hill et al., 2022; Leggat-Barr et al., 2021; Magesh et al., 2021) The potential role of effective therapeutics was a salient consideration in a pandemic characterized by a concerning level of vaccine hesitancy. Understanding the dynamic interplay between vaccine and treatment access and acceptance will be important for modeling uptake scenarios for smallpox MCMs.

While the nature and amounts of MCMs procured and stockpiled influence national infectious disease preparedness, comprehensive readiness necessitates a whole-of-society approach. The success of an MCM intervention rests on the successful delivery of the product and on sufficient uptake among target or prioritized populations. COVID-19 revealed in stark terms that social, ethical, political, and market factors are all part of the fabric of readiness and resilience. It is especially concerning that several U.S. states have taken actions to limit vaccination requirements, which weakens the capacity of the public health system or the federal government to respond to future viral threats (National Academy for State Health Policy, 2024).

An operational or implementation research agenda could be invaluable in developing an improved understanding and better planning for smallpox MCM deployment. Components of such a research agenda might include developing strategies for rapidly collecting real-world evidence, improving turnaround times for testing, and equity-related parameters. This information could be critical to appropriate stockpile planning.

Vaccine Hesitancy and Risk Communications

While it is outside the scope of the committee's charge to fully deliberate on the sociopolitical and economic factors that might influence stockpile decisions, the committee would like to highlight a few key dynamics that federal and state planners should consider in their decisions about smallpox readiness planning as they relate to downstream operational challenges.

Vaccine hesitancy is not a new phenomenon, but the national experience with COVID-19 and mpox demonstrated what vaccine hesitancy can mean for outbreak or pandemic response and how politics, policies, and misinformation can influence vaccine uptake. Planners must factor the potential role of vaccine hesitancy and other forms of mistrust of science, scientists, government, and industry into the predicted success of any smallpox strategy and seriously consider whether people will accept the risks associated with a replication-competent vaccine (see Chapter 1). Multiple studies have attempted to ascertain end-user acceptance of replicating smallpox vaccine. One study assessed health care provider willingness in 2002 to receive pre-event smallpox vaccination; 73 percent were willing, and the most common reason cited for those who did not want the vaccine was concern over adverse events (Everett et al., 2003). A second similar study yielded comparable results (Yih et al., 2003). But hesitance to receive the vaccine in the past (and today) may be related to the fact that smallpox is not in active circulation so it is reasonable to consider that uptake willingness might differ in a post-outbreak scenario. A 2004 analysis of differential willingness within the general public to undergo smallpox vaccination found that 84 percent of respondents reported being willing to get vaccinated in a hypothetical post-exposure ring vaccination scenario, and that number held regardless of racial identification; in a pre-exposure scenario, the number was substantially higher in White participants (77 percent) than African American (54 percent) (Micco et al., 2004).

What all of this indicates is that communicating the risk and benefits of smallpox vaccination versus infection, which carries far higher rates of disfiguration or death than does vaccination, will be critically important. But in the cases of COVID-19 and mpox, effective risk communication has been a struggle, especially in countering vaccine hesitancy driven by misinformation and disinformation about vaccines and the politicization of vaccination. These same challenges could occur in a smallpox outbreak and may be exasperated by other factors such as the origin of the small-pox event (e.g. laboratory accident or bioterror event) and who might be implicated in such an event (e.g., non-state actors or the laboratories that maintain the remaining live variola viruses in the United States and Russia). And while social and traditional media platforms will be able to quickly share images of smallpox patients from the 1960s and 1970s—showing the severity of the disease and hopefully encouraging intended populations to take protective measures—these same platforms could be used by actors to also propagate misinformation, disinformation, and altered imagery. Lessons learned about addressing misinformation, such as by enlisting locally trusted messengers, following public health risk communication principles (e.g., CDC's Crisis and Emergency Risk Communication program) and misinformation management strategies (CDC, 2018; Nagar et al., 2024), and learning from previous smallpox vaccine campaigns (IOM, 2005), could be critical to an effective risk communication response. Prepositioned statements and guidelines for smallpox prevention and treatment, including discussion about which interventions will likely be ineffective, could also be considered.

CDC has sample smallpox alert messages available on its website for state and local health departments to reference, but today these messages say only that smallpox is a "serious, life-threatening disease," with no further information about smallpox morbidity and mortality (CDC, 2017b). Variables that might affect uptake will include individual- and population-level willingness to receive vaccine; the level of risk messaged to the public; whether the vaccine is being administered pre- or post-exposure; the level of tolerance for vaccine side effects (especially because there are known severe adverse events of replicating smallpox vaccine); the dosing regimen (one versus two doses); and acceptance of old versus new vaccine technologies. Historical lessons from smallpox, polio, and measles vaccination campaigns, for example, show that vaccine hesitancy can be diminished when trusted community leaders guide vaccination efforts, individuals feel invested in vaccine development, and vaccination efforts are integrated with broader public health efforts (Eddy et al., 2023). Recent experiences with mpox highlight issues around vaccine hesitancy, access and availability, and disease stigma (Agroia et al., 2023; Mektebi et al., 2024; Moawad et al., 2023). Community anxiety and mental health implications of a disease outbreak and the public health response could also affect vaccine uptake and other health-related behaviors (Serafini et al., 2020) Overall, the public health community must gain the public trust by communicating clearly about the benefits, risks, and uncertainties in the deployment of vaccines and other MCMs.

Access to and uptake of COVID-19 countermeasures and concomitant health outcomes were often drawn along sociodemographic lines. Combinations of such factors as mistrust, geographic, financial, and cultural barriers to access, and language barriers led to differential access to and uptake of COVID MCMs by different ethnic, racial, geographic, political and other groups (Abba-Aji et al., 2022; Hill et al., 2022). These differences often led to starkly different health outcomes, stratified along racial, ethnic, and socioeconomic lines (Magesh et al., 2021). The wealth of studies on these dynamics can inform smallpox planning efforts and improve understanding about the:

- root causes of MCM hesitancy and how to evaluate and implement strategies to address hesitancy and how vaccine hesitancy relates to therapeutic hesitancy,
- role of transparency and science literacy in building trust in advance,
- role of avoiding or mitigating financial conflicts of interest in research on MCM development and production (IOM, 2009a), and
- planning for and anticipating public uptake based on the lessons learned from COVID-19 and mpox vaccine hesitancy and misinformation impacts (WHO, 2022).

Frontline Readiness and Biosafety

The COVID-19 and mpox experiences showed the importance of ensuring those on the front line—health care providers, public health practitioners and laboratorians, and first responders—have the capabilities and capacities to effectively and equitably diagnose, prevent, and treat in the event of an infectious disease outbreak. Jurisdictions must be prepared to receive vaccines, maintaining cold chain protocols, and preparing to repackage and further distribute (Adams, 2023).

According to IOM (2005), preparing key responders for smallpox does not necessarily involve vaccinating responders, but would ideally involve receive timely training and education to meet the demands of the situation. As mentioned in Chapter 2, smallpox is a disease that few clinicians in practice today have ever seen, and pox-like, lesion-causing diseases can be difficult to distinguish from each other (e.g., chickenpox and mpox have been mistaken for each other on initial evaluation, and one might expect similar initial confusion in a smallpox outbreak) (Leung, 2019).

Clinician readiness today requires sustaining a suspicion for the possibility of smallpox in patients with fever and a rash who test negative for other common pathogens. Once a single case is detected however, very rapid and intense engagement with the clinical community would be critical, including around diagnostic testing criteria and to provide up-to-date knowledge of the correct techniques for specimen collection and submission. The scope of clinician involvement would be related to the breadth of the outbreak. A small outbreak from an unintentional event, such as a lab accident, would be more contained and require a limited engagement of the local health care workforce and activation of appropriate regional or national quarantine and isolation facilities. An intentional release in a major population center, by contrast, would be a major health security event of immediate international concern, requiring mobilization across the health care system and the need to increase national and international readiness for possible further attacks. A large-scale national response would likely arise even if the initial number of cases were to be relatively limited, as illustrated by the U.S. response to the 2001 Anthrax letter attacks and the 2014–2016 Ebola cases. Furthermore, ongoing and intense engagement with clinicians, health systems, and first responders would be critical for optimizing public uptake of medical countermeasures, as noted above.

Since there are currently no point-of-care tests for smallpox, clinical recognition of smallpox among health care professionals will be extremely important during an outbreak. CDC has clinical guidance and evaluation flow charts available on its website (CDC, 2016, 2017a). Notably, CDC advises that health care providers use only personnel who have been vaccinated against smallpox to administer smallpox vaccines and to vaccinate exposed personnel within 72 (though preferably within 24) hours of their first exposure to a confirmed smallpox patient (CDC, 2017a). ASPR has indicated that shipping of smallpox MCMs from the SNS will begin within 8 hours after receiving the direction to deploy (Adams, 2023).

Clinical guidance for smallpox MCMs would need to be communicated to frontline providers. For example, the administration of replicating smallpox vaccine requires a multiple puncture technique that is different from that of other vaccines, and those who might need to deliver the vaccines may not be trained in this technique. Absent the application of this technique, the vaccine-neutralizing antibody titer mounted is minimal. The method, although easy to learn, causes pause for some clinicians, as it necessitates the appearance of blood spots where the bifurcated needle is used. A national program to train vaccinators in this technique at the local level would need to be rapidly implemented in the event of a smallpox outbreak, taking lessons from the national smallpox vaccination campaign that took place 2002–2003 (IOM, 2005). The most recent clinical guidance for smallpox vaccine use was published nearly a decade ago in 2015 and only provides guidance for a post-event vaccination program (Petersen et al., 2015). This guidance should be updated to reflect new data on smallpox vaccines—especially data about use for prevention of mpox and its efficacy—and clinical guidelines for indications and use of smallpox therapeutics should be developed. For example, frontline providers would also need rapid, situation-based training on the use of replicating and non-replicating vaccines and other updated clinical use guidance.

Strict and comprehensive biosafety measures must also be in place to manage a smallpox emergence, but there are only a handful of locations in the United States certified and equipped to intake smallpox patients (i.e., the National Special Pathogen System), and these would likely be rapidly overwhelmed in a large outbreak. Rapid training on special pathogen handling at facilities in an outbreak location would therefore be necessary. Even then, it is unclear whether testing facilities and the health care system would have the capacity to manage smallpox samples and patients safely and securely. In this regard, investments in developing strategies and infrastructure to carry out rapid regional trainings for outbreak response would improve smallpox (and other pathogen) preparedness. The nation's laboratory system should also be prepared to process smallpox samples. Opportunities to strengthen national laboratory systems based on experience from recent public health emergencies are described in Box 3-3. CDC reports that Laboratory Response Network (LRN) sites could be expanded to perform variola-specific testing if confirmatory testing is needed on a larger scale. As discussed in Chapter 2, diagnostics assays for variola are only available at select LRN labs due to biosafety considerations. This could result in low testing capacity at the beginning of a smallpox outbreak, not unlike the testing experiences at the start of COVID-19 and mpox in the United States. Smallpox is designated as a biosafety level 4 agent, so only a select number of laboratories could safely and securely process smallpox assays during the beginning of an outbreak. Furthermore, the LRN testing algorithm for smallpox is complex, and better suited for the detection of initial cases in the absence of smallpox than situations where disease is more established or widespread (King, 2023). WHO manages the biosafety inspections for the laboratories working with variola, which must comply with strict biosafety regulations (WHO, 2024b). In the event of a larger outbreak, an approach to expanding testing sites would have to take into consideration clinician recognition and familiarity with disease presentations, availability of potential technological advances including testing platforms or inactivation methods that allow tests to be performed at lower biosafety levels, increased biosafety and biosecurity training, and greater input from regulatory authorities regarding approval and certification processes (see below). Box 3-3 discusses potential solutions for smallpox testing issues.

BOX 3-3
Opportunities to Strengthen National
Laboratory Systems for Smallpox

Biosafety
- Collaborating with commercial laboratories for specimen transport during public health emergencies.[a]

Test Development
- Providing redundancy in the initial test development process using advanced public health laboratories.[a]

Test Manufacturing
- Proactively developing government contracts with test manufacturers for supplies.[a]

Stockpiling
- Robustly stocking the Strategic National Stockpile with testing kits, test components, and other related supplies.[b]

Testing Capacity
- Updating current LRN assays by multiplexing and adapting to high throughput.[*]
- Establishing guidelines to ensure consistency and predictability among traditional and nontraditional health care testing settings.[b]
- Striving toward immediate access to validated methods, the ability to rapidly develop methods, and a trained testing workforce.[b]
- Securing federal testing capacity by designating laboratories, medical centers and test manufacturers to respond during outbreaks.[c]
- Establishing emergency funding mechanisms before outbreaks can greatly impact mobilization efforts and testing readiness.[c]

Data Management
- Developing a minimum dataset for the test request process and case definition.[a]
- Standardizing laboratory information management systems to ensure data can be shared within the national laboratory system.[b]

Regulatory
- Collaborating with FDA to develop a portfolio of pre-vetted test protocols to speed regulatory test approval in an emerging biological crisis.[a]
- Aspiring toward nationwide mandatory reporting requirements to coordinate mitigation efforts.[b]
- Need for federal testing guidelines with enforcement and guidance structures.[b]
- Creating and updating test protocols that are pre-reviewed by FDA could speed regulatory test approvals during public health emergencies.[c]

BOX 3-3 Continued

Overall
- Collaborating across public and private fields to address current deficits in laboratory systems and ensure that rapid scale-up of testing is possible during large-scale emergencies.[b]
- Coordinating and advancing testing preparation across public health laboratories, hospitals, academic medical centers, commercial laboratories, health care providers, and patients is necessary in order to optimize capacities and contributions.

NOTES: Source attribution indicated by the following:
   [a]King (2023).
   [b]NASEM (2023).
   [c]Brown Pandemic Center (2023).
SOURCES: Brown Pandemic Center (2023); King (2023); NASEM (2023).

Drawing on information gathered by the committee and lessons from the testing experiences for COVID-19 and mpox, Box 3-3 lists opportunities for improving smallpox laboratory testing.

Regulatory Readiness

As noted in Chapter 1, access to smallpox MCMs in both domestic and global stockpiles depends considerably on the regulatory status of existing and new MCMs as well as on risk–benefit calculations that must be carried out with incomplete information. As such, these regulatory decisions reflect important scientific, legal, and ethical considerations. The success of a regulatory system in approving new drugs or new indications depends on the regulators' capacity, and recent reports have shown that FDA and its international partners struggle to keep pace with new products and applications (NASEM, 2020a,b). Furthermore, global regulatory and legal capacity must also be sufficient to approve safe and effective MCMs quickly and efficiently in the event of a smallpox outbreak.

Regulatory readiness must take into account two intertwined elements: timeliness and the ability to expand. Both COVID and mpox revealed that a timely early response can be enabled by the availability of diverse products, including vaccines, diagnostics, and therapeutics. A rapid and agile regulatory response to approving or otherwise authorizing promising MCMs can also support timelines. For the ability to expand—that is, to scale up manufacturing and the capacity to deliver those finished products to end users—public, private, and academic partners are necessary. Part of government readiness for MCMs is recognizing the importance of inclusion of other partners in virtually every aspect of preparedness. Supply chain issues are inevitable, for example, and if there are limited vendors for a particular MCM and there are quality issues, then downstream effects will be significant.

Regulatory decisions about the development and potential stockpiling and use of agents that have not yet been rigorously tested for safety and efficacy must balance multiple considerations. For instance, novel smallpox MCMs cannot be tested in humans with smallpox because the disease has been eradicated, but the use of MCMs developed for smallpox in the mpox outbreaks provided valuable proxy data indicating that they might have pan-orthopoxvirus applications (Dalton et al., 2023). There will always be some uncertainty about the cross-utility of MCMs within a viral family, but other orthopoxvirus outbreaks are considerably more likely than a smallpox outbreak, and investments in therapeutics targeting other orthopoxviruses might make it even more likely that these MCMs will have multiple uses and more immediate health benefits (i.e., will certainly be useful for other orthopoxvirus and might also be useful for smallpox).

At the point when a novel MCM is being developed and deployed, there is often a need to balance an understandable desire for rapid access to a promising new drug with ensuring that robust evidence is collected to determine if the product is in fact sufficiently safe and effective. Allowing an ineffective or harmful MCM to be deployed could raise false hopes of mitigation or, worse, cause significant harm to patients and whole populations. Yet delaying or disallowing authorization or approval of promising drugs until they are fully vetted would withhold potential benefits, especially for patients at greatest risk. Adhering to rigorous research ethics is essential even in the midst of a health emergency. In responding to COVID-19, for example, there has often been tension between providing rapid access (framed around respect for autonomy, "right to try," or "compassionate use") and conducting rigorous research to ensure that initially promising COVID MCMs are, in fact, safe and effective (Dominus, 2020). Efforts to navigate the competing values of rapid access versus rigorous research during the COVID-19 pandemic led, for example, to the initiation of platform trials in which every enrolled patient received a promising therapeutic (no one received placebo) (Macleod and Norrie, 2021). It also led to reassessments of the relative value of ongoing real-world evidence collection and strategies to improve the quality of this form of evidence as means of achieving this difficult balance (Schad and Thronicke, 2022).

These experiences from COVID-19 should be considered in planning for rapid MCM development, testing, and deployment in the event of a smallpox or other orthopoxvirus outbreak. For instance, the immediate initiation of a platform trial to compare the effectiveness of available proposed smallpox MCMs could lead to very rapid determinations of real-world effectiveness, which could be facilitated by having a research protocol in place and approved prior to the event.

Key MCM Regulations for Smallpox Readiness and Response

Under section 564 of the Federal Food, Drug, and Cosmetic Act[3], FDA may authorize unapproved medical products or uses during a public health emergency as declared by the Secretary of HHS under *Emergency Use Authorization* (EUA). All the COVID-19 vaccines were initially distributed under an EUA while their sponsors sought full approval. MVA-BN received FDA approval in 2019 for the prevention of smallpox and monkeypox disease in adults at high risk of infection. In 2022, however, faced with the realities of an outbreak that differed from the assumptions of the approval, FDA issued an EUA that expanded the population to those under 18 and permitted an alternate route of injection for adults (FDA, 2022a). Thus, while the SNS holds FDA-approved vaccines and treatments, an outbreak might necessitate the issuance of an EUA or an investigational new drug (IND) permit to use these in a different way. Such regulatory mechanisms could also enable the use of other products such as the Aventis Pasteur smallpox vaccine (see Chapter 2), which lacks FDA approval and would only be released under an EUA or IND "for use in circumstances where ACAM2000 is depleted, not readily available, or in a case-by-case basis where ACAM2000 is contraindicated" (CDC, 2022).

The emergency use of an unapproved investigational drug or biologic may require an IND (FDA, 1998). Emergency use is defined as the use of an investigational drug or biological product with a human subject in a life-threatening situation in which no standard acceptable treatment is available and in which there is not sufficient time to obtain institutional review board approval.[4] As of this writing, tecovirimat may be requested for mpox patients under an expanded access IND (CDC, 2024).

Expiration dating extension. Expiration dates of stockpiled MCMs can present challenges, and FDA is engaged in four approaches to extend expiration dates: initiated by the manufacturer, the shelf-life extension program, emergency use authorities, and enforcement discretion (FDA, 2024a). In February 2023, FDA approved a shelf-life extension for tecovirimat, a drug approved for smallpox and contained in the SNS, from 24 months to 42 months (FDA, 2024a).

Animal Rule. To prove the efficacy of a product during circumstances in which human challenge studies would not be ethical or feasible, such as for smallpox, FDA may grant approval based on well-controlled animal studies

---

[3] 21 U.S.C. § 360bbb-3.
[4] 21 CFR 56.102(d).

and demonstration of the product's safety in humans (FDA, 2023a). For example, tecovirimat was approved under FDA's Animal Rule after showing effectiveness and efficacy only in in vitro and animal model studies, coupled with safety data in humans (CDC, 2021).

Regulatory flexibility. Two federal regulations apply to laboratory testing for clinical use. The Clinical Laboratory Improvement Amendments regulate all laboratory testing (except research) performed on humans in the United States and it is overseen by the Centers for Medicare & Medicaid Services (CMS) (CMS, 2024). The second is the Food, Drug, and Cosmetic Act (FD&C) that applies to tests marketed for clinical use and is under FDA's jurisdiction. CMS and FDA may exercise enforcement discretion for diagnostics authorized under a public health emergency (e.g., enforcement discretion was applied during COVID-19, so tests could be run on asymptomatic individuals, which went beyond authorization limited to symptomatic individuals). Early in the COVID-19 pandemic, emergency provisions in the FD&C were invoked, giving FDA the ability to grant EUAs for diagnostic tests prior to completing the normal review process. This allowed many commercially developed tests to be available faster to the consumer. However, the same provisions simultaneously introduced additional requirements for laboratory developed tests (LDTs) requiring sites, such as hospitals and universities, to obtain an EUA for their home-grown tests (FDA, 2022b; Sluzala and Haislmaier, 2022). FDA has generally exercised enforcement discretion over LDTs, which waived pre-market review requirements needed on commercially marketed diagnostic tests. The FDA stance was further articulated during the mpox pandemic, when the agency reverted to enforcement discretion policies for certain mpox tests developed by laboratories, as long as the LDTs were performed in a high complexity Clinical Laboratory Improvement Amendments (CLIA)-certified lab, and were not at-home tests or did not include home specimen collection (FDA, 2023b).This allowed LDTs for mpox to be used at non-LRN sites (i.e., clinical or academic centers) increasing the number of patient testing sites and bringing testing closer to the patient (Caldera et al., 2023; Conger, 2022, FDA, 2023b). Recently, FDA, with support from CMS, has signaled that it will move away from its historic enforcement discretion stance and provide more oversight of LDTs (FDA, 2024b). Further clarification from FDA and CMS on how they will approach regulatory flexibility during future public health emergencies will be important factors in expanding access to testing and mitigating a smallpox outbreak of significant scale.

Relevant Ethical Questions for Smallpox MCMs

Basic science research on smallpox may fit the definition of dual use research of concern and therefore receives additional ethical scrutiny (NASEM, 2017). MCM research, by contrast, typically does not pose a direct dual use threat, insofar as research on or stockpiling of a new therapeutic or vaccine would not entail learning about how to make the virus more virulent or infectious. But developing and stockpiling MCMs does pose a closely related ethical challenge. Namely, adversaries might consider U.S. plans to vaccinate or treat the populace as a threat in that it would reduce U.S. vulnerability to a smallpox bioweapon. U.S. scientists and public health planners might view as unlikely the potential for the United States to develop and use a smallpox bioweapon in breach of its legal and ethical obligations, but planners should not assume all actors would have such reservations and others might not trust the United States to hold to its commitments. For this reason, strong and verifiable international agreements about resource and knowledge sharing, international collaborations, and transparency all hold special importance in the arena of smallpox MCM development and stockpiling.

Conclusions on Factors that Influence Readiness and Response Posture

(3-6) The small number of manufacturers of smallpox MCMs is a readiness and response vulnerability—and it is clear there is insufficient capacity to scale MCM production in the event of a large-scale smallpox event especially one of international scope.

(3-7) Given the lack of commercially available orthopoxvirus diagnostics, vaccines, and therapeutics, planning for logistics and supply chain management considerations is critical. Efforts could give consideration to developing plans to increase the number of smallpox vaccine and therapeutics manufacturers as well as optimizing current manufacturing capacities should they be needed in the shorter term.

(3-8) Communicating the risk and benefits of smallpox vaccination versus infection will be critically important. But experience with COVID-19 and mpox demonstrated that effective risk communication has been a challenge, especially considering vaccine hesitancy and the politicization of vaccination, and misinformation and disinformation. These same challenges could occur in a smallpox outbreak.

(3-9) Implementation research investigating the operational and social aspects of deploying and uptake of smallpox MCMs is needed to assess operational parameters that could affect readiness and response.

(3-10) Those on the front line—health care providers, public health practitioners and laboratorians, and first responders—need to have the capabilities and capacities to effectively and equitably diagnosis, prevent, and treat in the event of a smallpox outbreak. Clinical and public health guidance should be updated to reflect new data and new MCMs and should take into consideration the range of response strategies beyond post-exposure programs (i.e., ring vaccination).

(3-11) Regulatory readiness and responsiveness, applicable to all types of MCMs, will be critical in the event of a smallpox outbreak. This is especially relevant considering the additional laboratory biosafety concerns for smallpox compared with other orthopoxviruses.

(3-12) New regulatory models that can quickly evaluate MCMs that use novel platforms and newer methodologies need to be developed and implemented. This could be achieved through the sharing of necessary product characteristics, detailed submission requirements, and setting accepted benchmarks and immune assays (in the case of vaccines) ahead of time, as well as planning for surge staffing to ensure timely review and real-time engagement for inquiries.

OVERARCHING CONCLUSIONS

Based on the evidence and findings on the ongoing utility of orthopoxvirus research more broadly for smallpox readiness and response, on the implications of scientific and technological advancements on available smallpox MCMs, and on operational considerations affecting SNS planning, the committee drew the following overarching conclusions:

In addition to smallpox readiness, research should continue to be used to enhance readiness and response for other orthopoxviruses, this includes supporting the validation, approval and licensure, and commercialization of existing and next-generation MCMs for use in the management of non-variola orthopoxviruses as an efficient way to expand readiness more broadly by enabling vendor-managed inventory approaches to stockpiling.

A comprehensive and ongoing risk–benefit analysis is needed for smallpox MCMs research using emerging technologies as well as ongoing careful oversight to mitigate the risks of this research and ensure the risk–benefit balance is maintained.

Readiness and response efforts involving MCMs are complex due to many factors. MCM development, stockpiling, and distribution planning must be flexible, adaptable, and robust against multiple potential smallpox event scenarios. Planning strategies should account for the complexities of each scenario and aim to support several health and well-being outcomes (e.g., health, justice, equity, and national/international demand).

REFERENCES

Abba-Aji, M., D. Stuckler, S. Galea, and M. McKee. 2022. Ethnic/racial minorities' and migrants' access to COVID-19 vaccines: A systematic review of barriers and facilitators. *Journal of Migration and Health* 5:100086.

Adams, S. A. 2023. Strategic National Stockpile smallpox medical countermeasures overview. Presentation at Meeting 3 of the Committee on Current State of Research, Development, and Stockpiling of Smallpox MCMs of the National Academies. December 14. https://www.nationalacademies.org/event/41411_12-2023_meeting-3-of-the-committee-on-the-current-state-of-research-development-and-stockpiling-of-smallpox-medical-countermeasures (accessed February 18, 2024).

Agroia, H., E. Smith, A. Vaidya, S. Rudman, and M. Roy. 2023. Monkeypox (mpox) vaccine hesitancy among mpox cases: A qualitative study. *Health Promotion Practices* December 15:15248399231215054.

Alaska Department of Health. 2024. *Alaskapox virus.* https://health.alaska.gov/dph/Epi/id/Pages/Alaskapox.aspx (accessed January 22, 2024).

Antheia. 2024. Antheia completes successful product validation. *PR Newswire,* https://www.prnewswire.com/news-releases/antheia-completes-successful-product-validation-302026695.html (accessed February 5, 2024).

Antinori, S., G. Casalini, A. Giacomelli, and A. J. Rodriguez-Morales. 2023. Update on mpox: A brief narrative review. *InfezMed* 31(3):269–276.

Baylor, N. W., and J. L. Goodman. 2022. Vaccine preparedness for the next influenza pandemic: A regulatory perspective. *Vaccines (Basel)* 10(12):2136.

Berche, P. 2022. Life and death of smallpox. *La Presse Médicale* 51(3):104117.

Bolislis, W. R., M. L. de Lucia, F. Dolz, R. Mo, M. Nagaoka, H. Rodriguez, M. L. Woon, W. Yu, and T. C. Kühler. 2021. Regulatory agilities in the time of COVID-19: Overview, trends, and opportunities. *Clinical Therapeutics* 43(1):124–139.

Bray, M., and M. Buller. 2004. Looking back at smallpox. *Clinical Infectious Diseases* 38(6):882–889.

Breman, J. G., and D. A. Henderson. 2002. Diagnosis and management of smallpox. *New England Journal of Medicine* 346(17):1300–1308.

Broad, W. J., and J. Miller. 2002. Traces of terror: The bioterror threat; report provides new details of Soviet smallpox accident. *The New York Times,* June 15.

Brown Pandemic Center. 2023. *Testing playbook for biological emergencies.* Providence, RI: Brown University.

Burrell, C. J., C. R. Howard, and F. A. Murphy. 2017. Chapter 16: Poxviruses. In C. J. Burrell, C. R. Howard and F. A. Murphy (eds.), *Fenner and White's medical virology (5th edition).* London: Academic Press. Pp. 229–236.

Caldera, J. R., H. K. Gray, O. B. Garner, and S. Yang. 2023. FDA trial regulation of laboratory developed tests (LDTs): An academic medical center's experience with mpox in-house testing. *Journal of Clinical Virology* 169:105611.

Carlin, E. P., N. Giller, and R. Katz. 2017. Estimating the size of the U.S. population at risk of severe adverse events from replicating smallpox vaccine. *Public Health Nursing* 34(3):200–209.

Carlson, R. 2015. *Synthesis.* http://www.synthesis.cc/synthesis/2015/05/brewing_bad_biosecurity_policy (accessed March 2, 2024).

CDC (U.S. Centers for Disease Control and Prevention). 2003. Update: Multistate outbreak of monkeypox—Illinois, Indiana, Kansas, Missouri, Ohio, and Wisconsin, 2003. *Morbidity and Mortality Weekly Report* 52(27):642–646.

CDC. 2016. *Evaluating patients for smallpox.* https://www.cdc.gov/smallpox/clinicians/algorithm-protocol.html (accessed February 6, 2024).

CDC. 2017a. *Protect and care for smallpox patients.* https://www.cdc.gov/smallpox/bioterrorism-response-planning/healthcare-facility/protect-care-patients.html (accessed February 6, 2024).

CDC. 2017b. *Sample alert messages for the community.* https://www.cdc.gov/smallpox/bioterrorism-response-planning/public-health/sample-alert-messages-community.html (accessed February 12, 2024).

CDC. 2018. *Crisis & Emergency Risk Communication (CERC).* https://emergency.cdc.gov/cerc (accessed February 28, 2024).

CDC. 2021. *Treatment.* https://www.cdc.gov/smallpox/clinicians/treatment.html (accessed February 7, 2024).

CDC. 2022. *Vaccines.* https://www.cdc.gov/smallpox/clinicians/vaccines.html (accessed February 7, 2024).

CDC. 2023. *COVID data tracker.* https://covid.cdc.gov/covid-data-tracker/#datatracker-home (accessed February 28, 2024).

CDC. 2024. *Tecovirimat (TPOXX) for treatment of mpox.* https://www.cdc.gov/poxvirus/mpox/clinicians/obtaining-tecovirimat.html (accessed February 12, 2024).

Chaplin, P. 2023. Current state of research, development, and stockpiling of smallpox MCMs. Presentation at Meeting 3 of the Committee on Current State of Research, Development, and Stockpiling of Smallpox MCMs of the National Academies. December 14. https://www.nationalacademies.org/event/41411_12-2023_meeting-3-of-the-committee-on-the-current-state-of-research-development-and-stockpiling-of-smallpox-medical-countermeasures (accessed February 18, 2024).

Chen, Y. E., D. Bousbaine, A. Veinbachs, K. Atabakhsh, A. Dimas, V. K. Yu, A. Zhao, N. J. Enright, K. Nagashima, Y. Belkaid, and M. A. Fischbach. 2023. Engineered skin bacteria induce antitumor T cell responses against melanoma. *Science* 380(6641):203–210.

CMS (Centers for Medicare & Medicaid Services). 2024. *Clinical Laboratory Improvement Amendments (CLIA).* https://www.cms.gov/medicare/quality/clinical-laboratory-improvement-amendments (accessed February 15, 2024).

Conger, K. 2022. *Mpox test launched at Stanford Medicine to help combat global outbreak.* https://med.stanford.edu/news/all-news/2022/06/monkeypox-test.html (accessed February 29, 2024).

Cooper, R. M., J. A. Wright, J. Q. Ng, J. M. Goyne, N. Suzuki, Y. K. Lee, M. Ichinose, G. Radford, F. J. Ryan, S. Kumar, E. M. Thomas, L. Vrbanac, R. Knight, S. L. Woods, D. L. Worthley, and J. Hasty. 2023. Engineered bacteria detect tumor DNA. *Science* 381(6658):682–686.

Costa, T., M. F. Stidworthy, R. Ehmann, D. Denk, I. Ashpole, G. Drake, I. Maciuca, G. Zoeller, H. Meyer, and J. Chantrey. 2023. Cowpox in zoo and wild animals in the United Kingdom. *Journal of Comparative Pathology* 204:39–46.

Dalton, A. F., A. O. Diallo, A. N. Chard, D. L. Moulia, N. P. Deputy, A. Fothergill, I. Kracalik, C. W. Wegner, T. M. Markus, P. Pathela, W. L. Still, S. Hawkins, A. T. Mangla, N. Ravi, E. Licherdell, A. Britton, R. Lynfield, M. Sutton, A. P. Hansen, G. S. Betancourt, J. V. Rowlands, S. J. Chai, R. Fisher, P. Danza, M. Farley, J. Zipprich, G. Prahl, K. A. Wendel, L. Niccolai, J. L. Castilho, D. C. Payne, A. C. Cohn, and L. R. Feldstein. 2023. Estimated effectiveness of jynneos vaccine in preventing mpox: A multijurisdictional case-control study—United States, August 19, 2022–March 31, 2023. *Morbidity and Mortality Weekly Report* 72(20):553–558.

Damon, I. K., C. R. Damaso, and G. McFadden. 2014. Are we there yet? The smallpox research agenda using variola virus. *PLOS Pathogens* 10(5):e1004108.

Decker, M. D., P. M. Garman, H. Hughes, M. A. Yacovone, L. C. Collins, C. D. Fegley, G. Lin, G. DiPietro, and D. M. Gordon. 2021. Enhanced safety surveillance study of ACAM2000 smallpox vaccine among US military service members. *Vaccine* 39(39):5541–5547.

Dobrovolná, M., V. Brázda, E. F. Warner, and S. Bidula. 2023. Inverted repeats in the monkeypox virus genome are hot spots for mutation. *Journal of Medical Virology* 95(1):e28322.

DoD (Department of Defense). 2020. *DOD approves $87 million for newest bioindustrial manufacturing innovation institute.* Washington, DC: Department of Defense.

Dominus, S. 2020. The COVID drug wars that pitted doctor vs. doctor. *The New York Times Magazine,* August 5. https://www.nytimes.com/2020/08/05/magazine/covid-drug-wars-doctors.html (accessed February 7, 2024).

Durski, K. N., A. M. McCollum, Y. Nakazawa, B. W. Petersen, M. G. Reynolds, S. Briand, M. H. Djingarey, V. Olson, I. K. Damon, and A. Khalakdina. 2018. Emergence of monkeypox—West and Central Africa, 1970–2017. *Morbidity and Mortality Weekly Report* 67(10):306–310.

Eddy, J. J., H. A. Smith, and J. E. Abrams. 2023. Historical lessons on vaccine hesitancy: Smallpox, polio, and measles, and implications for COVID-19. *Perspectives in Biology and Medicine* 66(1):145–159.

Esparza, J., S. Lederman, A. Nitsche, and C. R. Damaso. 2020. Early smallpox vaccine manufacturing in the United States: Introduction of the "animal vaccine" in 1870, establishment of "vaccine farms", and the beginnings of the vaccine industry. *Vaccine* 38(30):4773–4779.

Everett, W. W., S. E. Coffin, T. Zaoutis, S. D. Halpern, and B. L. Strom. 2003. Smallpox vaccination: A national survey of emergency health care providers. *Academic Emergency Medicine* 10(6):606–611.

FDA (U.S. Food and Drug Administration). 1998. *Emergency use of an investigational drug or biologic: Guidance for institutional review boards and clinical investigators.* https://www.fda.gov/regulatory-information/search-fda-guidance-documents/emergency-use-investigational-drug-or-biologic (accessed February 7, 2024).

FDA. 2022a. *Fact sheet for healthcare providers administering vaccine: Emergency Use Authorization of JYNNEOS (smallpox and monkeypox vaccine, live, non-replicating) for prevention of monkeypox disease in individuals determined to be at high risk for monkeypox infection.* https://www.fda.gov/media/160774/download (accessed February 15, 2024).

FDA. 2022b. *Policy for monkeypox tests to address the public health emergency: Guidance for laboratories, commercial manufacturers and Food and Drug Administration staff.* https://www.fda.gov/regulatory-information/search-fda-guidance-documents/policy-monkeypox-tests-address-public-health-emergency (accessed March 2, 2024).

FDA. 2023a. *Animal rule information.* https://www.fda.gov/emergency-preparedness-and-response/mcm-regulatory-science/animal-rule-information (accessed February 15, 2024).

FDA. 2023b. *Monkeypox (mpox) and medical devices.* https://www.fda.gov/medical-devices/emergency-situations-medical-devices/monkeypox-mpox-and-medical-devices#Laboratories (accessed February 6, 2024).

FDA. 2024a. *Expiration dating extension.* https://www.fda.gov/emergency-preparedness-and-response/mcm-legal-regulatory-and-policy-framework/expiration-dating-extension#mpoxsmallpox (accessed February 15, 2024).

FDA. 2024b. *FDA and CMS: Americans deserve accurate and reliable diagnostic tests, wherever they are made.* https://www.fda.gov/medical-devices/medical-devices-news-and-events/fda-and-cms-americans-deserve-accurate-and-reliable-diagnostic-tests-wherever-they-are-made (accessed March 2, 2024).

GAO (Government Accountability Office). 2021. *Science & tech spotlight: Genomic sequencing of infectious pathogens (GAO-21-426SP).* Washington, DC: Government Accountability Office.

GAO. 2022. *HHS and DOD transitioned vaccine responsibilities to HHS, but need to address outstanding issues (GAO-22-104453).* Washington, DC: Government Accountability Office.

GAO. 2023. *Public health preparedness: HHS should plan for medical countermeasure development and manufacturing risks (GAO-23-105713).* Washington, DC: Government Accountability Office.

Gong, Q., C. Wang, X. Chuai, and S. Chiu. 2022. Monkeypox virus: A re-emergent threat to humans. *Virologica Sinica* 37(4):477–482.

Grabenstein, J. D., and W. Winkenwerder, Jr. 2003. U.S. military smallpox vaccination program experience. *JAMA* 289(24):3278–3282.

Grad, Y. H., and M. Lipsitch. 2014. Epidemiologic data and pathogen genome sequences: A powerful synergy for public health. *Genome Biology* 15(11):538.

Gubser, C., S. Hué, P. Kellam, and G. L. Smith. 2004. Poxvirus genomes: A phylogenetic analysis. *Journal of General Virology* 85(1):105–117.

Hammarlund, E., M. W. Lewis, S. G. Hansen, L. I. Strelow, J. A. Nelson, G. J. Sexton, J. M. Hanifin, and M. K. Slifka. 2003. Duration of antiviral immunity after smallpox vaccination. *Nature Medicine* 9(9):1131–1137.

Hedberg, H., and A. Zink. 2024. *Fatal Alaskapox infection in a Southcentral Alaska resident.* State of Alaska Epidemiology Bulletin. https://epi.alaska.gov/bulletins/docs/b2024_02.pdf (accessed February 15, 2024).

Hepburn, M. 2023. Remarks on lessons learned and future considerations for smallpox prepared-ness and readiness. Presentation at Meeting 3 of the Committee on Current State of Research, Development, and Stockpiling of Smallpox MCMs of the National Academies. December 14. https://www.nationalacademies.org/event/41411_12-2023_meeting-3-of-the-committee-on-the-current-state-of-research-development-and-stockpiling-of-smallpox-medical-countermeasures (accessed February 18, 2024).

HHS (Department of Health and Human Services). 2010. *Screening framework guidance for providers of synthetic double-stranded DNA.* https://www.phe.gov/Preparedness/legal/guidance/syndna/Documents/syndna-guidance.pdf (accessed February 15, 2024).

Hill, L., S. Artiga, A. Rouw, and J. Kates. 2022. How equitable is access to COVID-19 treatments? *KFF,* June 23. https://www.kff.org/coronavirus-covid-19/issue-brief/how-equitable-is-access-to-covid-19-treatments (accessed February 15, 2024).

Hoffmann, S. A., J. Diggans, D. Densmore, J. Dai, T. Knight, E. Leproust, J. D. Boeke, N. Wheeler, and Y. Cai. 2023. Safety by design: Biosafety and biosecurity in the age of synthetic genomics. *iScience* 26(3):106165.

Impelluso, G., and F. Lentzos. 2017. The threat of synthetic smallpox: European perspectives. *Health Security* 15(6):582–586.

IOM (Institute of Medicine). 2005. *The smallpox vaccination program: Public health in an age of ter-rorism.* Washington, DC: The National Academies Press.

IOM. 2009a. *Conflict of interest in medical research, education, and practice.* Washington, DC: The National Academies Press.

IOM. 2009b. *Live variola virus: Considerations for continuing research.* Washington, DC: The National Academies Press.

Jacobs, B. L., J. O. Langland, K. V. Kibler, K. L. Denzler, S. D. White, S. A. Holechek, S. Wong, T. Huynh, and C. R. Baskin. 2009. Vaccinia virus vaccines: Past, present and future. *Antiviral Research* 84(1):1–13.

Jaschke, P. R., G. A. Dotson, K. S. Hung, D. Liu, and D. Endy. 2019. Definitive demonstration by synthesis of genome annotation completeness. *Proceedings of the National Academy of Sciences* 116(48):24206–24213.

Jauneikaite, E., K. S. Baker, J. G. Nunn, J. T. Midega, L. Y. Hsu, S. R. Singh, A. L. Halpin, K. L. Hopkins, J. R. Price, P. Srikantiah, B. Egyir, I. N. Okeke, K. E. Holt, S. J. Peacock, and N. A. Feasey. 2023. Genomics for antimicrobial resistance surveillance to support infection prevention and control in health-care facilities. *The Lancet Microbe* 4(12):e1040–e1046.

Jezek, Z., and F. Fenner. 1988. Human monkeypox. Vol. 17 in *Monographs in virology.* S.Karger AG.

Jiang, T., G. Li, R. Liu, J. Zhou, N. Gao, and J. Shen. 2023. Creating an ultra-sensitive detection platform for monkeypox virus DNA based on CRISPR technology. *Journal of Medical Virology* 95(7):e28905.

Kaminski, M. M., O. O. Abudayyeh, J. S. Gootenberg, F. Zhang, and J. J. Collins. 2021. CRISPR-based diagnostics. *Nature Biomedical Engineering* 5(7):643–656.

Kates, J., J. Tolbert, and A. Rouw. 2002. *The red/blue divide in COVID-19 vaccination rates continues: An update.* https://www.kff.org/policy-watch/the-red-blue-divide-in-covid-19-vaccination-rates-continues-an-update (accessed February 28, 2024).

Kennedy, R. B., and P. A. Gregory. 2023. Chapter 55 - smallpox and vaccinia. In *Plotkin's vaccines (eighth edition),* edited by W. Orenstein, P. Offit, K. M. Edwards and S. Plotkin. Philadelphia: Elsevier. Pp. 1057–1086.

King, E. 2023. Lessons learned and future considerations for smallpox preparedness and readiness. Presentation at Meeting 3 of the Committee on Current State of Research, Development, and Stockpiling of Smallpox MCMs of the National Academies. December 14. https://www.nationalacademies.org/event/41411_12-2023_meeting-3-of-the-committee-on-the-current-state-of-research-development-and-stockpiling-of-smallpox-medical-countermeasures (accessed February 18, 2024).

Kuiken, T. 2023. *Artificial intelligence in the biological sciences: Uses, safety, security, and oversight.* Washington, DC: Congressional Research Service.

Leggat-Barr, K., N. Goldman, and F. Uchikoshi. 2021. COVID-19 risk factors and mortality among Native Americans. *Demographic Research* 45(39):1185–1218.

Leung, J., A. M. McCollum, K. Radford, C. Hughes, A. S. Lopez, S. A. J. Guagliardo, B. Nguete, T. Likafi, J. Kabamba, J. Malekani, R. Shongo Lushima, E. Pukuta, S. Karhemere, J. J. Muyembe Tamfum, M. G. Reynolds, E. Wemakoy Okitolonda, D. S. Schmid, and M. Marin. 2019. Varicella in Tshuapa Province, Democratic Republic of Congo, 2009–2014. *Tropical Medicine & International Health* 24(7):839–848.

Levrier, A., I. Karpathakis, B. Nash, S. D. Bowden, A. B. Lindner, and V. Noireaux. 2023. Pheiges, all-cell-free phage synthesis and selection from engineered genomes. *bioRxiv* 2023.2012.2007.570578.

Liu, J., S. Wennier, L. Zhang, and G. McFadden. 2011. M062 is a host range factor essential for myxoma virus pathogenesis and functions as an antagonist of host SAMD9 in human cells. *Journal of Virology* 85(7):3270–3282.

Macleod, J., and J. Norrie. 2021. PRINCIPLE: A community-based COVID-19 platform trial. *The Lancet Respiratory Medicine* 9(9):943–945.

Magesh, S., D. John, W. T. Li, Y. Li, A. Mattingly-app, S. Jain, E. Y. Chang, and W. M. Ongkeko. 2021. Disparities in COVID-19 outcomes by race, ethnicity, and socioeconomic status: A systematic review and meta-analysis. *JAMA Network Open* 4(11):e2134147.

Martín-Acebes, M. A., N. Jiménez de Oya, and J. C. Saiz. 2019. Lipid metabolism as a source of druggable targets for antiviral discovery against zika and other flaviviruses. *Pharmaceuticals (Basel)* 12(2):97.

Massung, R. F., L.-I. Liu, J. Qi, J. C. Knight, T. E. Yuran, A. R. Kerlavage, J. M. Parsons, J. C. Venter, and J. J. Esposito. 1994. Analysis of the complete genome of smallpox variola major virus strain Bangladesh–1975. *Virology* 201(2):215–240.

Mayes, C. 2023. CRISPR-based antivirals as broad-spectrum therapeutics. Presentation at Meeting 3 of the Committee on Current State of Research, Development, and Stockpiling of Smallpox MCMs of the National Academies. December 14. https://www.nationalacademies.org/event/41411_12-2023_meeting-3-of-the-committee-on-the-current-state-of-research-development-and-stockpiling-of-smallpox-medical-countermeasures (accessed February 18, 2024).

McInnes, C. J., I. K. Damon, G. L. Smith, G. McFadden, S. N. Isaacs, R. L. Roper, D. H. Evans, C. R. Damaso, O. Carulei, L. M. Wise, and E. J. Lefkowitz. 2023. ICTV virus taxonomy profile: Poxviridae 2023. *Journal of General Virology* 104(5). https://doi.org/10.1099/jgv.0.001849 (accessed March 2, 2024).

Mektebi, A., M. Elsaid, T. Yadav, F. Abdallh, M. Assker, A. Siddiq, R. Sayad, M. Saifi, and R. A. Farahat. 2024. Mpox vaccine acceptance among healthcare workers: A systematic review and meta-analysis. *BMC Public Health* 24(1):4.

Micco, E., A. D. Gurmankin, and K. Armstrong. 2004. Differential willingness to undergo smallpox vaccination among African-American and White individuals. *Journal of General Internal Medicine* 19(5 Pt 1):451–455.

Moss, B., and G. L. Smith. 2021. Chapter 16: *Poxviridae*: The viruses and their replication. In P. M. Howley and D. M. Knipe (eds.), *Fields virology: DNA viruses, vol. 2 (7th edition)*. Philadelphia: Wolters Kluwer Health. Pp. 573–613.

Moawad, M. H.-E., A. M. Taha, D. Nguyen, M. Ali, Y. A. Mohammed, W. A. E.-T. Moawad, E. Hamouda, D. K. Bonilla-Aldana, and A. J. Rodriguez-Morales. 2023. Attitudes towards receiving monkeypox vaccination: A systematic review and meta-analysis. *Vaccines* 11(12):1840.

Mouton, C. A., C. Lucas, and E. Guest. 2023. *The operational risks of AI in large-scale biological attacks: A red-team approach*. Santa Monica, CA: RAND Corporation.

Mutz, P., W. Resch, G. Faure, T. G. Senkevich, E. V. Koonin, and B. Moss. 2023. Exaptation of inactivated host enzymes for structural roles in orthopoxviruses and novel folds of virus proteins revealed by protein structure modeling. *mBio* 14(2):e0040823.

Nagar, A., V. Grégoire, A. Sundelson, E. O'Donnell-Pazderka, A. M. Jamison, and T. K. Sell. 2024. *Practical playbook for addressing health misinformation*. Baltimore, MD: Johns Hopkins Center for Health Security.

NASEM (National Academies of Sciences, Engineering, and Medicine). 2016. *Global health risk framework: Research and development of medical products: Workshop summary*. Washington, DC: The National Academies Press.

NASEM. 2017. *Dual use research of concern in the life sciences: Current issues and controversies.* Washington, DC: The National Academies Press.

NASEM. 2020a. *Regulating medicines in a globalized world: The need for increased reliance among regulators.* Washington, DC: The National Academies Press.

NASEM. 2020b. *Stronger food and drug regulatory systems abroad.* Washington, DC: The National Academies Press.

NASEM. 2021. *Ensuring an effective public health emergency medical countermeasures enterprise.* Washington, DC: The National Academies Press.

NASEM. 2022a. *Building resilience into the nation's medical product supply chains.* Washington, DC: The National Academies Press.

NASEM. 2022b. *Globally resilient supply chains for seasonal and pandemic influenza vaccines.* Washington, DC: The National Academies Press.

NASEM. 2023. *Future of the nation's laboratory systems for health emergency response: Proceedings of a workshop—in brief.* Washington, DC: The National Academies Press.

National Academy for State Health Policy. 2024. *State efforts to limit or enforce COVID-19 vaccine mandates.* https://nashp.org/state-tracker/state-efforts-to-ban-or-enforce-covid-19-vaccine-mandates-and-passports (accessed February 7, 2024).

Ndodo, N., J. Ashcroft, K. Lewandowski, A. Yinka-Ogunleye, C. Chukwu, A. Ahmad, D. King, A. Akinpelu, C. Maluquer de Motes, P. Ribeca, R. P. Sumner, A. Rambaut, M. Chester, T. Maishman, O. Bamidele, N. Mba, O. Babatunde, O. Aruna, S. T. Pullan, B. Gannon, C. S. Brown, C. Ihekweazu, I. Adetifa, and D. O. Ulaeto. 2023. Distinct monkeypox virus lineages co-circulating in humans before 2022. *Nature Medicine* 29(9):2317–2324.

Nguyen, E., M. Poli, M. G. Durrant, A. W. Thomas, B. Kang, J. Sullivan, M. Y. Ng, A. Lewis, A. Patel, A. Lou, S. Ermon, S. A. Baccus, T. Hernandez-Boussard, C. Ré, P. D. Hsu, and B. L. Hie. 2024. Sequence modeling and design from molecular to genome scale with Evo. *bioRxiv* 2024.2002.2027.582234.

Ninove, L., Y. Domart, C. Vervel, C. Voinot, N. Salez, D. Raoult, H. Meyer, I. Capek, C. Zandotti, and R. N. Charrel. 2009. Cowpox virus transmission from pet rats to humans, France. *Emerging Infectious Diseases* 15(5):781–784.

Nou, X. A., and C. A. Voigt. 2024. Sentinel cells programmed to respond to environmental DNA including human sequences. *Nature Chemical Biology* 20(2):211–220.

Noyce, R. S., S. Lederman, and D. H. Evans. 2018. Construction of an infectious horsepox virus vaccine from chemically synthesized DNA fragments. *PLOS One* 13(1):e0188453.

NTI (Nuclear Threat Initiative). 2024. *New international biosecurity organization launched to safeguard bioscience.* https://www.nti.org/news/new-international-biosecurity-organization-launched-to-safeguard-bioscience (accessed February 29, 2024).

O'Toole, Á., R. A. Neher, N. Ndodo, V. Borges, B. Gannon, J. P. Gomes, N. Groves, D. J. King, D. Maloney, P. Lemey, K. Lewandowski, N. Loman, R. Myers, I. F. Omah, M. A. Suchard, M. Worobey, M. Chand, C. Ihekweazu, D. Ulaeto, I. Adetifa, and A. Rambaut. 2023. APOBEC3 deaminase editing in mpox virus as evidence for sustained human transmission since at least 2016. *Science* 382(6670):595–600.

Parrino, J., and B. S. Graham. 2006. Smallpox vaccines: Past, present, and future. *Journal of Allergy and Clinical Immunology* 118(6):1320–1326.

Pastoret, P. P., and A. Vanderplasschen. 2003. Poxviruses as vaccine vectors. *Comparative Immunology, Microbiology, & Infectious Diseases* 26(5–6):343–355.

Peng, C., S. L. Haller, M. M. Rahman, G. McFadden, and S. Rothenburg. 2016. Myxoma virus M156 is a specific inhibitor of rabbit PKR but contains a loss-of-function mutation in Australian virus isolates. *Proceedings of the National Academy of Sciences* 113(14):3855–3860.

Perdiguero, B., P. Pérez, L. Marcos-Villar, G. Albericio, D. Astorgano, E. Álvarez, L. Sin, C. E. Gómez, J. García-Arriaza, and M. Esteban. 2023. Highly attenuated poxvirus-based vaccines against emerging viral diseases. *Journal of Molecular Biology* 435(15):168173.

Petersen, B. W., and I. K. Damon. 2015. 136: Other poxviruses that infect humans: Parapoxviruses (including orf virus), molluscum contagiosum, and yatapoxviruses. In J. E. Bennett, R. Dolin and M. J. Blaser (eds.), *Mandell, Douglas, and Bennett's principles and practice of infectious diseases (8th edition)*. Philadelphia: W.B. Saunders. Pp. 1703–1706.

Petersen, B. W., I. K. Damon, C. A. Pertowski, D. Meaney-Delman, J. T. Guarnizo, R. H. Beigi, K. M. Edwards, M. C. Fisher, S. E. Frey, R. Lynfield, and R. E. Willoughby. 2015. Clinical guidance for smallpox vaccine use in a postevent vaccination program. *Morbidity and Mortality Weekly Report Recommendations and Reports* 64(2):1–32.

Petersen, B. W., T. J. Harms, M. G. Reynolds, and L. H. Harrison. 2016. Use of vaccinia virus smallpox vaccine in laboratory and health care personnel at risk for occupational exposure to orthopoxviruses—Recommendations of the Advisory Committee on Immunization Practices (ACIP), 2015. *Morbidity and Mortality Weekly Report* 65(10):257–262.

Qin, D. 2019. Next-generation sequencing and its clinical application. *Cancer Biology & Medicine* 16(1):4–10.

Reardon, S. 2014. Infectious diseases: Smallpox watch. *Nature* 509(7498):22–24.

Reynolds, M. G., W. B. Davidson, A. T. Curns, C. S. Conover, G. Huhn, J. P. Davis, M. Wegner, D. R. Croft, A. Newman, N. N. Obiesie, G. R. Hansen, P. L. Hays, P. Pontones, B. Beard, R. Teclaw, J. F. Howell, Z. Braden, R. C. Holman, K. L. Karem, and I. K. Damon. 2007. Spectrum of infection and risk factors for human monkeypox, United States, 2003. *Emerging Infectious Diseases* 13(9):1332–1339.

Robinson, P. C., D. F. L. Liew, H. L. Tanner, J. R. Grainger, R. A. Dwek, R. B. Reisler, L. Steinman, M. Feldmann, L. P. Ho, T. Hussell, P. Moss, D. Richards, and N. Zitzmann. 2022. COVID-19 therapeutics: Challenges and directions for the future. *Proceedings of the National Academy of Sciences* 119(15):e2119893119.

Sandbrink, J. B. 2023 (unpublished). Artificial intelligence and biological misuse: Differentiating risks of language models and biological design tools. *arXiv* https://doi.org/10.48550/arXiv.2306.13952.

Satheshkumar, P. S., and I. K. Damon. 2021. Chapter 17: Poxviruses. In P. M. Howley and D. M. Knipe (eds.), *Fields virology: DNA viruses, vol. 2 (7th edition)*. Philadelphia: Wolters Kluwer Health. Pp. 614–640.

Schad, F., and A. Thronicke. 2022. Real-world evidence—current developments and perspectives. *International Journal of Environmental Research and Public Health* 19(16):10159.

Serafini, G., B. Parmigiani, A. Amerio, A. Aguglia, L. Sher, and M. Amore. 2020. The psychological impact of COVID-19 on the mental health in the general population. *QJM* 113(8):531–537.

Shao, B. 2024. A long-context language model for the generation of bacteriophage genomes. *bioRxiv* 2023.2012.2018.572218.

Sinclair, C. 2023. About emergent. Presentation at Meeting 3 of the Committee on Current State of Research, Development, and Stockpiling of Smallpox MCMs of the National Academies. December 14. https://www.nationalacademies.org/event/41411_12-2023_meeting-3-of-the-committee-on-the-current-state-of-research-development-and-stockpiling-of-smallpox-medical-countermeasures (accessed February 18, 2024).

Sluzala, Z., and E. Haislmaier. 2022. *Lessons from COVID-19: How policymakers should reform the regulation of clinical testing*. https://www.heritage.org/public-health/report/lessons-covid-19-how-policymakers-should-reform-the-regulation-clinical/#_ftnref9 (accessed March 2, 2024).

Smith, G. L., C. T. O. Benfield, C. Maluquer de Motes, M. Mazzon, S. W. J. Ember, B. J. Ferguson, and R. P. Sumner. 2013. Vaccinia virus immune evasion: Mechanisms, virulence and immunogenicity. *Journal of General Virology* 94(11):2367–2392.

Srinivasan, P., and C. D. Smolke. 2020. Biosynthesis of medicinal tropane alkaloids in yeast. *Nature* 585(7826):614–619.

Taub, D. D., W. B. Ershler, M. Janowski, A. Artz, M. L. Key, J. McKelvey, D. Muller, B. Moss, L. Ferrucci, P. L. Duffey, and D. L. Longo. 2008. Immunity from smallpox vaccine persists for decades: A longitudinal study. *American Journal of Medicine* 121(12):1058–1064.

Thi Nhu Thao, T., F. Labroussaa, N. Ebert, P. V'Kovski, H. Stalder, J. Portmann, J. Kelly, S. Steiner, M. Holwerda, A. Kratzel, M. Gultom, K. Schmied, L. Laloli, L. Hüsser, M. Wider, S. Pfaender, D. Hirt, V. Cippà, S. Crespo-Pomar, S. Schröder, D. Muth, D. Niemeyer, V. M. Corman, M. A. Müller, C. Drosten, R. Dijkman, J. Jores, and V. Thiel. 2020. Rapid reconstruction of SARS-CoV-2 using a synthetic genomics platform. *Nature* 582(7813):561–565.

Torres-Domínguez, L. E., and G. McFadden. 2019. Poxvirus oncolytic virotherapy. *Expert Opinion on Biological Therapy* 19(6):561–573.

Tucker, J. B. 2002. *Scourge: The once and future threat of smallpox.* Grove Press.

Upton, C., S. Slack, A. L. Hunter, A. Ehlers, and R. L. Roper. 2003. Poxvirus orthologous clusters: Toward defining the minimum essential poxvirus genome. *Journal of Virology* 77(13):7590–7600.

Van Dijck, C., N. A. Hoff, P. Mbala-Kingebeni, N. Low, M. Cevik, A. W. Rimoin, J. Kindrachuk, and L. Liesenborghs. 2023. Emergence of mpox in the post-smallpox era—A narrative review on mpox epidemiology. *Clinical Microbiology and Infection* 29(12):1487–1492.

Warfel, K. F., A. Williams, D. A. Wong, S. E. Sobol, P. Desai, J. Li, Y. F. Chang, M. P. DeLisa, A. S. Karim, and M. C. Jewett. 2023. A low-cost, thermostable, cell-free protein synthesis platform for on-demand production of conjugate vaccines. *ACS Synthetic Biology* 12(1):95–107.

White House. 2023. *Executive order on the safe, secure, and trustworthy development and use of artificial intelligence, October 30, 2023.* https://www.whitehouse.gov/briefing-room/presidential-actions/2023/10/30/executive-order-on-the-safe-secure-and-trustworthy-development-and-use-of-artificial-intelligence (accessed February 29, 2024).

WHO (World Health Organization). 2015. *The Independent Advisory Group on Public Health Implications of Synthetic Biology Technology Related to Smallpox, June 2015.* https://www.who.int/publications/i/item/the-independent-advisory-group-on-public-health-implications-of-synthetic-biology-technology-related-to-smallpox (accessed February 15, 2024).

WHO. 2022. Understanding the behavioural and social drivers of vaccine uptake: WHO position paper, May 2022. *Weekly Epidemiological Record* 97:209–224.

WHO. 2023a. *Mpox (monkeypox)—Democratic Republic of the Congo.* November 23. https://www.who.int/emergencies/disease-outbreak-news/item/2023-DON493 (accessed December 22, 2023).

WHO. 2023b. *Multi-country outbreak of mpox, external situation report #31—22 December.* https://www.who.int/publications/m/item/multi-country-outbreak-of-mpox--external-situation-report-31---22-december-2023 (accessed February 15, 2024).

WHO. 2023c. *WHO Advisory Committee on Variola Virus Research: Report of the twenty-fourth meeting, Geneva, 29–30 November 2022.* https://www.who.int/publications/i/item/9789240076310 (accessed February 28, 2024).

WHO. 2024a. *154th session of the executive board, provisional agenda item 18—Smallpox eradication: Destruction of variola virus stocks (January 2).* https://apps.who.int/gb/ebwha/pdf_files/EB154/B154_20-en.pdf (accessed February 15, 2024).

WHO. 2024b. *Variola virus repository safety inspections.* https://www.who.int/activities/variola-virus-repository-safety-inspections (accessed February 4, 2024).

WHO Executive Board. 2024. *Intervention by the delegate of the Russian Federation.* 154th Session, Agenda Item 18. January 25. https://www.who.int/about/accountability/governance/executive-board/executive-board-154th-session (accessed February 28, 2024).

Yezli, S., and J. A. Otter. 2011. Minimum infective dose of the major human respiratory and enteric viruses transmitted through food and the environment. *Food and Environmental Virology* 3(1):1–30.

Yih, W. K., T. A. Lieu, V. H. Rêgo, M. A. O'Brien, D. K. Shay, D. S. Yokoe, and R. Platt. 2003. Attitudes of healthcare workers in U.S. hospitals regarding smallpox vaccination. *BMC Public Health* 3:20.

Yinka-Ogunleye, A., O. Aruna, D. Ogoina, N. Aworabhi, W. Eteng, S. Badaru, A. Mohammed, J. Agenyi, E. N. Etebu, T.-W. Numbere, A. Ndoreraho, E. Nkunzimana, Y. Disu, M. Dalhat, P. Nguku, A. Mohammed, M. Saleh, A. McCollum, K. Wilkins, O. Faye, A. Sall, C. Happi, N. Mba, O. Ojo, and C. Ihekweazu. 2018. Reemergence of human monkeypox in Nigeria, 2017. *Emerging Infectious Diseases* 24(6):1149–1151.

Yuan, S., H. Chu, J. F.-W. Chan, Z.-W. Ye, L. Wen, B. Yan, P.-M. Lai, K.-M. Tee, J. Huang, D. Chen, C. Li, X. Zhao, D. Yang, M. C. Chiu, C. Yip, V. K.-M. Poon, C. C.-S. Chan, K.-H. Sze, J. Zhou, I. H.-Y. Chan, K.-H. Kok, K. K.-W. To, R. Y.-T. Kao, J. Y.-N. Lau, D.-Y. Jin, S. Perlman, and K.-Y. Yuen. 2019. SREBP-dependent lipidomic reprogramming as a broad-spectrum antiviral target. *Nature Communications* 10(1):120.

Zhang, F., Q. Ji, J. Chaturvedi, M. Morales, Y. Mao, X. Meng, L. Dong, J. Deng, S. B. Qian, and Y. Xiang. 2023. Human SAMD9 is a poxvirus-activatable anticodon nuclease inhibiting codon-specific protein synthesis. *Science Advances* 9(23):eadh8502.

Zubair, M., J. Wang, Y. Yu, M. Faisal, M. Qi, A. U. Shah, Z. Feng, G. Shao, Y. Wang, and Q. Xiong. 2022. Proteomics approaches: A review regarding an importance of proteome analyses in understanding the pathogens and diseases. *Frontiers in Veterinary Science* 9:1079359.

4

Way Forward: Priorities for Research, Development, and Stockpiling

"In a smallpox emergency, a reemergence anywhere will likely create demand [for medical countermeasures] everywhere."
Crystal Watson, in presentation to the committee
December 14, 2023

Decades of investments have reaped significant benefits for smallpox preparedness, even if the threat of a smallpox outbreak is of uncertain size and scope. The United States now has a smallpox stockpile of medical countermeasures (MCMs) far more robust and mature than it was at its inception. The committee was asked to provide its perspective on what the priorities could be going forward for additional research, development, and the stockpiling of smallpox MCMs that can further improve the U.S. readiness and response posture. What knowledge gaps remain that could be addressed through scientific research, and what capability gaps remain that could be addressed through amendment to the composition of the stockpile? This chapter briefly discusses future opportunities for live variola virus research as well as for non-variola orthopoxvirus research in developing smallpox MCMs and concludes with considerations for new directions in the national stockpiling approach for smallpox MCMs.

SMALLPOX RESEARCH AGENDA

Research that enhances the safety, efficacy, and utility of smallpox diagnostics, vaccines, and therapeutics provides a public health benefit in the context of smallpox readiness and has added benefits that improve the nation's response to other orthopoxvirus outbreaks. Objectives to date of the U.S. smallpox research program derive largely from the 1999 Institute of Medicine (IOM) report that addressed the scientific needs for live variola virus (IOM, 1999) and subsequent reports of the IOM (IOM, 2009) and the World Health Organization (WHO) Advisory Group of Independent Experts (WHO, 2010, 2013) and have been overseen by the WHO Advisory Group for Live Variola Virus Research (ACVVR) (WHO, n.d.). Table 4-1 highlights conclusions from the 1999 and 2009 IOM reports and the 2022 ACVVR report (WHO, 2023). The 2023 ACVVR report (in progress at the time of publication) was recently summarized at the 154th WHO Executive Board Session and concluded that access to and use of live variola virus remains essential for public health needs, including completing the sequencing of remaining variola virus isolates, further research on point-of-care diagnostics, the development of scalable less-reactogenic vaccines, and the development of small-molecule antiviral agents (WHO, 2024a). Figure 4-1, from the U.S. Centers for Disease Control and Prevention (CDC), illustrates a U.S. smallpox research agenda focused on next-generation vaccines, antiviral treatments, and nucleic acid- and protein-based diagnostic assays and shows nodes at which variola viral samples enable the evaluation of the diagnostics, vaccines, and therapeutics developed under this agenda.

U.S. investments in line with this agenda have expanded the smallpox assets available to the United States (and to other countries). These investments have also enabled benefits beyond smallpox readiness and response. These benefits were realized most clearly in the mpox response's use of modified vaccinia Ankara-Bavarian Nordic (MVA-BN) and tecovirimat, countermeasures which at their inception were envisioned exclusively for smallpox preparedness. Inversely, one would expect a research program targeting non-variola orthopoxviruses to offer potential utility for smallpox preparedness and, further, that investments in products with broader and potentially commercial use may have more immediate utility and could be more attractive to industry partners. As discussed in Chapter 3, while orthopoxviruses in general offer great utilities, vaccinia virus, the prototype poxvirus and the smallpox vaccine, and the monkeypoxvirus are of particular significance in this regard. Both these viruses emerged as human pathogens post cessation of smallpox vaccination programs (Damaso et al., 2000).

Non-Variola Orthopoxvirus and Live Variola Virus Research

This section identifies gaps and opportunities in the discovery and development pipeline for smallpox MCMs and describes the ongoing role of the use of live variola virus. Research with live variola virus and with non-variola orthopoxviruses is necessary to the development of smallpox MCMs—leading to better diagnostics, better vaccines, and better

TABLE 4-1 List of Conclusions from the IOM Reports: *Assessment of Future Scientific Needs for Live Variola Virus* (1999) and *Live Variola Virus: Considerations for Continuing Research* (2009) and Recommendations from the 2022 ACVVR Report

Type of Research	Conclusions from the 1999 IOM Report	Conclusions from the 2009 IOM Report	Recommendations from the 2022 ACVVR Report
Diagnostics	If further development of procedures for the environmental detection of variola virus or for diagnostic purposes were to be pursued, more extensive knowledge of the genome variability, predicted protein sequences, virion surface structure, and functionality of variola virus from widely dispersed geographic sources would be needed.	Live variola virus is not required for further development of detection and diagnostic methods. Virus materials such as DNA and proteins would suffice for this purpose. *NOTE: The 2009 IOM report is in conflict with the ACVVR 2022 report in that live variola virus is required for the further development of detection and diagnostic methods. This reflects, lessons learned from past public health emergencies per the need for diagnostics which are readily available to triage decision making.	Continue work on roadmap to leverage advances in smallpox diagnostics for further development of point-of-care diagnostics for mpox. Continue to work toward development and validation of (rapid, point-of-care) orthopoxvirus diagnostic tests and expedite their availability in a reliable and equitable manner. Continue to work toward development of protein-based orthopoxvirus diagnostics with continuing focus on approaches that do not require the use of live variola virus, noting that development of nucleic acid–based diagnostics does not require the use of live variola virus. Consider development of target product profiles for smallpox diagnostics.

continued

TABLE 4-1 Continued

Type of Research	Conclusions from the 1999 IOM Report	Conclusions from the 2009 IOM Report	Recommendations from the 2022 ACVVR Report
Therapeutics	The most compelling reason for long-term retention of live variola virus stocks is their essential role in the identification and development of antiviral agents for use in anticipation of a large outbreak of smallpox. It must be emphasized that if the search for antiviral agents with activity against live variola virus were to be continued, additional public resources would be needed.	For both scientific and regulatory reasons, the final developmental stages leading to licensure of smallpox therapeutics cannot occur without the use of live variola virus. Furthermore, although the regulatory environment may change, the scientific reasons will remain. Therapeutic agents need to be evaluated against a representative panel of variola strains to reduce the possibility that some strains might be naturally resistant.	Continue development and discovery of small molecule antivirals for use by themselves or in combination to give maximal protection in case of a smallpox event and to delay or slow down the emergence of resistance. Continue work to identify genetic markers of resistance to antivirals.
Vaccines	Adequate stocks of smallpox vaccine must be maintained if research is to be conducted on variola virus or if maintenance of a smallpox vaccination program is required. Live variola virus would be necessary if certain approaches to the development of novel types of smallpox vaccine were pursued.	The current development and licensure pathway for first- and second-generation vaccinia vaccines that produce a "take" does not require use of the live variola virus. Use of the live virus will be necessary, however, for the development and licensure of any vaccine that does not manifest such a cutaneous lesion at the site of inoculation	Continue efforts to characterize the effectiveness against other orthopoxviruses of smallpox vaccines approved or in development, and support studies particularly against mpox in field settings. Continue work to characterize and harmonize potency testing protocols for all smallpox vaccines. Continue efforts to improve the shelf life of vaccines. Include minimally- or non-replicating vaccines in WHO strategic reserves.

Genomic Analysis	Genomic sequencing and limited study of variola surface proteins derived from geographically dispersed specimens is an essential foundation for important future work. Such research could be carried out now and could require a delay in the destruction of known stocks but would not necessitate their indefinite retention.	Live variola virus is not needed for variola genome sequence analysis if specimens containing viral DNA of adequate quantity and quality are available. Live variola virus would be needed for functional genomics–based experimental approaches.	Complete full genome sequencing of variola virus strains or isolates without amplification of virus and make sequence data for all available isolates publicly available directly or via WHO as soon as possible.
Animal Models	The existence of animal models would greatly assist the development and testing of antiviral agents and vaccines as well as studies of variola pathogenesis. Such a program could be carried out only with live variola virus.	That a comprehensive evaluation of the work done to date on the nonhuman primate model of variola pathogenesis be undertaken by CDC, in conjunction with an expert panel knowledgeable about poxviruses and animal models of viral infection. The objective would be to identify ways in which the predictive value of the model for diagnostics, therapeutics, and vaccines might be improved.	No recommendations made in this area
Discovery Research	Live or replication-defective variola virus would be needed if studies of variola pathogenesis were to be undertaken to provide information about the response of the human immune system. Variola virus proteins have potential as reagents in studies of human immunology. Live variola virus would be needed for this purpose only until sufficient variola isolates had been cloned and sequenced.	Discovery research to gain greater understanding of human physiology and immunology, while not essential, would require use of the live variola virus and might ultimately support efforts to discover and evaluate therapeutics and vaccines. Further, research with live variola virus and research with variola proteins could lead to discoveries with broader implications for human health.	Only addressed whether to continue current plans for MCM research

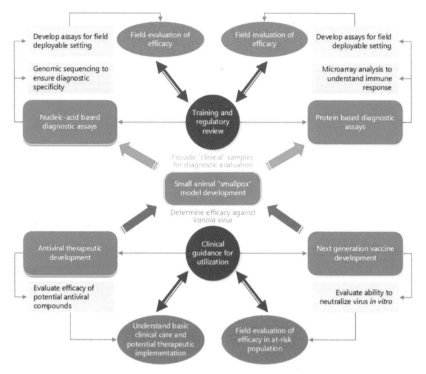

FIGURE 4-1 Smallpox research agenda.
SOURCE: Hutson (2023).

therapeutics. The necessary regulatory restrictions on research with live variola virus and the absence of circulating smallpox disease today make orthopoxvirus research using non-variola species critical to continued improvements in smallpox preparedness. Scientific and technological advancements in studying orthopoxviruses in humanized-mouse models, Cast E/J mice, other small animal models, nonhuman primate animal models, and in silico models have also created opportunities to complement the use of variola virus research (Hutson et al., 2021).

Non-Variola Orthopoxvirus Research

The following narrative lays out important advances in smallpox MCMs using non-variola orthopoxvirus research. Working with non-variola orthopoxviruses can inform new strategies and approaches for scaling and improving MCM production and distribution. U.S. Food and Drug Administration (FDA)-approved smallpox vaccines are formulated using vaccinia virus, a non-variola orthopoxvirus. All first-, second-, and third-generation smallpox vaccines contain vaccinia virus, an orthopoxvirus closely related to variola which has been proven to prevent most smallpox disease and deaths. In fact, the first-generation smallpox vaccine was labeled by FDA for "prevention of orthopoxvirus" disease, and the newest licensed smallpox vaccine, MVA-BN, is labeled for the prevention of both smallpox and mpox. Vaccinia research therefore has direct implications for vaccine safety, efficacy, shelf-life, improvement, production, cost reduction, and management. Additionally, mpox subunit and nucleic acid vaccines (including mRNA vaccines) in development are rooted in the understanding of other orthopoxviruses (Fang et al., 2023; Freyn et al., 2023; Hooper et al., 2003; Hou et al., 2023; Rcheulishvili et al., 2023; Sang et al., 2023; X. Yang et al., 2023; Zeng et al., 2023; Zhang et al., 2023).

Non-variola orthopoxviruses have also been used in the development and testing of smallpox drugs and can support future drug development for smallpox and other targets. Efforts to develop new therapeutics for smallpox have used non-variola orthopoxviruses in preclinical and clinical trials and have shown efficacy against them (Deng et al., 2007; Dower et al., 2012; Peng et al., 2020). The development processes of the smallpox drugs tecovirimat (Huggins et al., 2009; G. Yang et al., 2005) and brincidofovir (Olson et al., 2014; Stabenow et al., 2010) relied on experimentation with non-variola orthopoxviruses and supportive studies with variola virus. The scientific and logistical limitations of using smallpox virus in animal models necessitated establishing the efficacy of tecovirimat using related viruses. Tecovirimat use demonstrated benefit in a number of animal models (mice, prairie dogs, rabbits, nonhuman primates) that had been infected with different orthopoxviruses (ectromelia, monkeypox, rabbitpox) as well as nonhuman primates infected with smallpox virus (variola virus) (Russo et al., 2021). Recent studies demonstrated benefit of tecovirimat in the treatment of humanized mice infected with smallpox virus (WHO, 2023). Pivotal studies for regulatory approval used nonhuman primates challenged with monkeypox virus and rabbits with rabbitpox virus and demonstrated improved survival in animals that received the drug (FDA, n.d.).

Because the presence of non-variola orthopoxviruses in the world complicates empirical diagnosis of smallpox, it thereby necessitates a research approach to diagnostics that differentiates between variola and these other viruses. The high similarity of orthopoxvirus DNA genome sequences and the recognition of new viruses have also posed challenges for accurate differentiation among orthopoxviruses using tests based on biophysical properties and sometimes nucleic acid–based tests, though reliable polymerase chain reaction (PCR) assays have been developed and continue to be reassessed as new viruses are discovered (Altindis et al., 2022; Hedberg and Zink, 2024; Low et al., 2023; Stefano et al., 2023). To date, serology-based approaches are challenged to distinguish among orthopoxviruses due to cross reactivity. The development of two FDA-approved nucleic acid-based assays—one for variola and one for non-variola orthopoxviruses—was designed to address the need for effective testing tools and an algorithm with which to use them. Validation of the non-variola panel relied on use of human pathogenic orthopoxviruses including strains of cowpox, monkeypox, vaccinia, and variola virus species[1] (FDA, 2018; Li et al., 2006).

Not only is non-variola orthopoxvirus research important in smallpox MCMs, but this research can also help reveal to scientists the reservoirs, evolutionary relationships, and virological properties of the genus, all of which can inform scientific understanding of variola virus and strategies to mitigate it. And since these viruses exist in nature and some are the cause of occasional or ongoing outbreaks, research on non-variola orthopoxviruses has a greater potential for near-term clinical and public health benefits. Use of these poxviruses could drive basic research in other areas as well, such as the study of viral vectors for vaccine development, gene therapy, and oncolytic virus therapy, as described in Chapter 3.

Live Variola Virus Research

While there are advantages to conducting research with non-variola orthopoxviruses, these species cannot fully replace the knowledge gained by working with live variola virus (Damon et al., 2014). In a presentation to the committee, CDC shared salient examples of the ways that strains of variola virus (or samples derived from live virus) have been or are being used, which include:

- Validation of diagnostic assays and iterative assessment of Laboratory Response Network tests with newly sequenced variola virus isolates *in silico* to determine if wet lab testing is needed.
- Provision of comparative data on vaccine immunogenicity, such as an ongoing study to provide "non-inferiority" data on MVA-BN at the request of FDA.
- Provision of comparative data on antiviral effectiveness to test an expanded panel of variola virus isolates for their sensitivity to tecovirimat at the request of FDA (Hutson, 2023).

As mentioned in Chapter 1, WHO oversees all research using live variola virus, with the ACVVR reviewing all research proposals that request to use one of the two sanctioned collections of live virus at CDC in Atlanta and the Russian State Centre for Research on Virology and Biotechnology (VECTOR), Koltsovo, Novosibirsk Region, Russian Federation. Box 4-1 highlights completed and ongoing research for use of live variola virus from

---

[1] Variola virus was used in the testing panel to confirm the assay did not detect variola virus.

BOX 4-1
Research Program Using Live Variola Virus, 2020–2023

CDC

- Genomic sequencing: Completing genomic sequencing of 40 isolates
- Diagnostics: Adapting and optimizing multiplex nucleic acid diagnostic tests for new platforms and settings. Continuing development and optimization of protein-based tests
- Antivirals: Tecovirimat, ST-357, completing screens of monoclonal antibodies (mAbs) and antibody mixes to neutralize variola virus, assisting in creating a new universal orthopoxvirus monoclonal mix, evaluating mAbs and cocktails in vitro against variola virus
- Vaccines: Finalize efficacy testing on long-term titer samples from MVA-BN and/or LC16m8 vaccine trials (as samples are available)
- Animal models: Completing remaining in vitro work on humanized mouse models HU-BLT, continuing assessment of HU-BLT and HU-CD34 models using tecovirimat

VECTOR

- Genomic sequencing: Completing genomic sequencing of 50 of remaining 88 isolates
- Diagnostics: Optimizing design of immunochemistry test kit and its accessories using orthopoxviruses
- Antivirals: NIOCH-14 oral formulation, 15 new compounds found to be highly active against orthopoxviruses, evaluating antivirals against variola virus based on monoclonal antibodies
- Vaccine: VACdelta6 testing completed, licensure obtained in 2022 as OrthopoxVac for smallpox, mpox, and other orthopoxviruses

WHO Oversight

- Advisory Committee for Variola Virus Research established in 1999 to oversee live variola virus research in accordance with World Health Assembly Resolution WHA52
- Oversight of live variola virus research, biosafety and biosecurity of both repository sites, sequencing the viral genome from variola virus isolates, and distribution of live variola DNA to other researchers (WHO, 2024b)
- BSL-4 level laboratory biosafety security measures in place to restrict access to variola virus
- Regular inspections and emergency drills; biannual WHO inspections
- Annual submission of proposals to work with live variola virus reviewed by the WHO ACVVR

SOURCES: Hutson (2023); Lewis (2023).

2020 to 2023. The 2022 ACVVR report of the 24th meeting also details specific research proposals for use of live variola virus presented for 2023, and the forthcoming 2023 report of the 25th meeting will detail specific research proposals presented for 2024 (in progress at the time of publication).

Notably, the ACVVR reports also describe a considerable amount of work using non-variola orthopoxviruses as surrogates and as useful tools in their own right for non-variola diseases like mpox (WHO, 2023).

Despite considerable similarities in genetic identity, host range, transmission, pathogenesis, and other viral characteristics and host interactions, research reveals significant differences across orthopoxvirus species (Satheshkumar and Damon, 2021). It is believed that genes in the left and right ends of the genomes, which are more variable across orthopoxviruses and are described to interact with multiple host proteins (e.g., interferons, complement, apoptosis, chemokines), are responsible for these differences (Moss and Smith, 2021). The genomic sequencing of variola virus isolates held in CDC and VECTOR repositories (still in progress) can contribute to the understanding of poxvirus evolution, host-range, virulence, and transmission and to the future assessment and evaluation of diagnostic assays and modern molecular techniques for diagnostics, and identification of variants that may be resistant to future antiviral drugs (WHO, 2023). Additional work in genomic sequencing of live variola virus will be required to advance the fundamental understanding of smallpox and related poxviruses, and WHO has recommended that sequence data for all available isolates be made publicly available as soon as possible.

In 1999, IOM concluded:

> The most compelling need for long-term retention of live variola virus would be for the development of antiviral agents or novel vaccines to protect against a reemergence of smallpox due to accidental or intentional release of variola virus. (IOM, 1999)

IOM's 1999 finding that live virus is needed for certain aspects of research remains true today. Further elucidation of some of the secrets of variola virus that remain hidden—and which could help advance the development of modernized smallpox MCMs—would necessitate research with live variola. For example, having live variola virus collections, before treatment with tecovirimat, will be important for understanding drug resistant mutants when they arise. Taking what is now known, Table 4-2 looks at smallpox MCM readiness as a function of research with live variola and non-variola orthopoxviruses. It maps the potential for using these viruses or their components against specific knowledge gaps and MCM goals that could support improved public health benefit.

TABLE 4-2 Smallpox MCM Readiness as a Function of Live Variola and Non-Variola Viral Research: Opportunities for MCM Improvement

Note to reader: This table is designed to emphasize smallpox MCM and research, but other orthopoxviruses are integrated where appropriate to smallpox preparedness. Rather than emphasizing the maintenance of existing MCM and incremental improvements on them, it highlights areas where more significant innovation could improve public health readiness and response outcomes.

Element of MCM Readiness	Smallpox MCM	Knowledge	Viral Research			
	Opportunity for MCM Improvement	Knowledge Gaps and Research Possibilities	Non-VARV Orthopoxviruses	Replication-Defective VARV	Live VARV in Tissue Culture	Live VARV in Animal Models
Detection tools and diagnostics	• Multiplex nucleic acid assays for new platforms and field settings. • Forward-deployed point-of-care assays including protein- or antigen-based tests to rapidly test and isolate infected patients. • FDA-approved serologic assays to assess individual and population levels of immunity against smallpox and history of exposures. • Nucleic acid testing of clinical samples (e.g., nasopharyngeal, saliva, urine, etc.) to test for disease prior to onset of rash illness.	Increasing surveillance and sequencing of variola samples to provide new knowledge about viral science that can advance MCM science: • Orthopoxvirus ecology • Orthopoxvirus epidemiology • Orthopoxvirus/variola genomic evolution • Orthpoxvirus immune responses	*Useful* to *essential* depending on specific pathogens	*Useful* for certain variola detection or diagnostic devices	*Useful* for certain variola detection or diagnostic devices	Full genome sequence is required, and live VARV is *essential* for optimal verification of diagnostics

TABLE 4-2 Continued

Element of MCM Readiness	Opportunity for MCM Improvement	Knowledge Gaps and Research Possibilities	Non-VARV Orthopoxviruses	Replication-Defective VARV	Live VARV in Tissue Culture	Live VARV in Animal Models
Vaccines	• Vaccines against smallpox with improved efficacy, safety, utility, and scalability. • Ancillary benefits of vaccinia-based vaccines for use as oncolytic virotherapies, vaccine vectors, and gene deliveries to build population immunity against smallpox and other orthopoxviruses.	Advancing research on orthopoxvirus replication, pathogenesis, host interactions, and immune responses to improve understanding of virus and host features that can support improved vaccines: • Vaccine immune response mechanisms and durability • Viral protein functions and functional interactions • Major targets of neutralizing antibodies • Immunodominant antigens/epitopes • Host and viral elements that determine breakthrough infections	*Essential* for almost every aspect of vaccine development with vaccinia virus	*No use*	*Useful* for measuring functional immune response (e.g., neutralization)	*Arguably essential* for optimal verification of potential efficacy in humans

		Essential for development due to the restricted access to VARV	*No use*	*Essential* for some targets	*Essential* for optimal verification of the MCM that will be used in humans
Antivirals	• New drugs with different and diverse targets, mechanisms of action, and routes of administration. • Drug cocktail effect (combined treatment).	Studying basic orthopoxvirus processes to support new knowledge in basic orthopoxvirus science toward improved antivirals: • Viral evolution, including genomic mutations from orthopoxvirus patients • Transmission • Pathogenesis and host interaction • Mechanisms of entry and receptors, DNA replication, transcription, membrane assembly, virion assembly and egress, and resistance • Viral protein functions and functional interactions • Major targets of neutralizing antibodies • Factors that determine host range • Cellular mechanisms promoting zoonotic infection			

continued

TABLE 4-2 Continued

Element of MCM Readiness	Opportunity for MCM Improvement	Knowledge Gaps and Research Possibilities	Non-VARV Orthopoxviruses	Replication-Defective VARV	Live VARV in Tissue Culture	Live VARV in Animal Models
Non-vaccine biologics	• Potential to repurpose vaccinia immune globulin intravenous (VIGIV) as part of combination therapy. • Novel treatment concepts and development, e.g., genome editing, nonconventional targets. • Monoclonal antibodies and antibody cocktails.	Applying of new technology to basic poxvirus discovery research to support improved understanding of virus and host properties that can improve biologics development: • Orthopoxvirus replication, pathogenesis, transmission, and host interaction • Major targets of neutralizing antibodies Applying research tools to study orthopoxvirus-based vaccine vectors and oncolytic agents can support novel therapies.	*Essential* for development due to the restricted access to VARV	*No use*	May be *essential* if advanced organoid or other sophisticated systems will be used to study these biologic interventions	*Essential* optimal verification of MCM that will be used in humans
Animal models (as they relate to MCMs)	• Understanding of vaccine and therapeutic efficacy and utility.	Researching improved humanized mouse models using VARV that can recapitulate aspects of human smallpox to support advances in vaccines and treatments.	*Essential*	*No use*	*Useful* for propagation of virus for testing in the animal model system	*Essential* in developing models that can be used for MCM efficacy testing as a human surrogate

NOTE: VARV = variola virus.

Research Readiness

The ability to evaluate the safety and efficacy of MCMs (particularly those that have only animal data on efficacy) in a larger population during a public health emergency is a critical component of MCM readiness. Clinical trial infrastructure serves as the backbone for evaluating urgently needed diagnostics, vaccines, and therapeutics during outbreaks (NASEM, 2017).

Advancement of therapeutics for COVID-19 lagged behind the successes with vaccines because at the outset of the pandemic, when little was known about the virus, but hospitalization rates were high, it was important to determine if existing antiviral agents could be repurposed for use. This was initially successful with Remdesivir. Thereafter, the drug discovery was slow knowing that because direct acting antiviral treatments work best when given early in the course of most diseases to halt viral replication and to be initiated on treatment, patients or participants must have access to diagnostics to confirm the presence of disease (Griffin et al., 2021; Mulangu et al., 2019). While clinical trial networks enabled rapid recruitment for hospitalized and moderately to severely ill patients, some argued that the lack of an established framework outside of hospitalized patients to support clinical trials was a significant challenge for research on early/mild COVID that led to small, underpowered studies with repurposed drugs (Robinson et al., 2022). This meant that the trials that were run offered limited insight into pre- or post-hospital stages of COVID-19. The COVID-19 pandemic highlighted the need for adaptive and outpatient trial designs, including community or nursing home based as well cluster trials for early access to treatment and for evaluation of pre- and post-exposure interventions (Griffin et al., 2021; Mulangu et al., 2019). Decentralizing and taking clinical trials closer to the community has the potential to also reduce social inequities and logistical barriers in research participation (Petrini et al., 2022). Even hospital-based trials faced immense delays in initiation and were fraught with inequity in participation by diverse patient populations (Linas and Cunningham, 2019). Had the government established an organized network of hospitals for the execution of large clinical trials and rapid data sharing, some argued, science could have produced more answers and potentially more solutions for health care providers who faced a high burden of hospitalizations and deaths with very few therapeutic tools in the first year of the pandemic (Zimmer, 2021).

Delays in initiating and conducting clinical trials can translate to lost lives and prolonged control efforts. Goals 3 and 4 of the National Biodefense Strategy and Implementation Plan lay out the whole-of-society elements of a fast response, calling for expedited evaluation of novel vaccines, therapeutics, and diagnostics during outbreaks (White House, 2022). WHO also recognizes the value of rapid research in a crisis, stating that strengthening clinical trial capacity within and across countries is essential for the timely development and evaluation of countermeasures (WHO, 2022a).

Additionally, emerging infectious diseases often present unique challenges that require tailored or adaptive study designs and infrastructure. These may include limited knowledge of the pathogen, difficulty recruiting participants, and complex logistical hurdles in outbreak settings. The preplanning of trials can not only increase the speed of response but also provide time for necessary consideration of ethical and logistic hurdles as well as for developing a strategy for the inclusion of diverse patient populations. COVID-19 and mpox emergencies have illustrated the importance of:

- Pre-pandemic preparedness: Establishing networks of trained researchers and clinical sites ready to pivot to emerging threats.
- Streamlined and adaptive trial designs: Developing flexible and efficient trial designs suitable for outbreak settings that allow evaluation of interventions in all phases of disease and bring trials closer to the patient in the community.
- Enhanced recruitment strategies: Implementing community engagement and outreach to ensure diverse participation.
- Regulatory planning and agility: Creating a streamlined and anticipatory review and approval process for clinical protocols for investigational MCMs to address emerging threats and fostering collaboration between regulatory bodies for faster and more efficient evaluation and approval of promising interventions.

Conclusions on the Continued Role of Live Variola Virus for Research and Public Health Purposes

(4-1) Research with live variola virus is essential for developing animal models to be used for MCM efficacy testing as a human surrogate, full verification of the potential efficacy of MCMs, and the development of certain targets for more effective therapeutic options, and it may be essential if advanced organoid or other sophisticated systems will be used to study these biologic interventions.

(4-2) Discovery research and pathogenesis research with live variola virus has merit as biomedical research without an immediate obvious connection to smallpox readiness and response.

(4-3) It is important to plan for clinical trials (e.g., of vaccine comparative effectiveness in conjunction with therapeutics and diagnostic testing) that will take place under real-world conditions during a smallpox outbreak to ensure that the following are in place: adaptive and streamlined trial designs, efforts toward diverse and equitable patient participation, and regulatory protocols that have been preapproved.

STOCKPILING CONSIDERATIONS

The committee was asked to help the Administration for Strategic Preparedness and Response (ASPR) think about the future of the smallpox MCM portfolio for the U.S. Strategic National Stockpile (SNS). A smallpox outbreak of any size (even a single case) will be initially perceived as an event of national and possible international (pandemic) potential, and the SNS will need to be forward leaning in its response until the source and scope of the outbreak are clear.

Historically, the SNS has prioritized and devoted most of its resources to just two threats—smallpox and anthrax (GAO, 2022; Kuiken and Gottron, 2023). These threats remain substantive drivers of the SNS budget, and there is limited flexibility in terms of what other MCMs can be purchased with current appropriations, due to the portion of the budget allocated to anthrax and smallpox MCMs (GAO, 2022). The president's fiscal year (FY) 2024 budget request for the SNS is $995 million. The request does not delineate the specific products it intends to procure with these funds, but the most recent multi-year budget from the Public Health Emergency Medical Countermeasures Enterprise (PHEMCE) offers insight into how the dollars, if appropriated, are likely to be spent. The budget proposed by PHEMCE describes increased funding needs in FY 2024 driven largely by higher spending on the anthrax, Ebola, and smallpox portfolios (HHS, 2023). Over the course of the five-year budget plan (FY 2022–2026), "sustainment of Anthrax and Smallpox capacity is expected to account for approximately two-thirds of SNS's procurement budget." If these PHEMCE projections become reflected in future budgets, then anthrax and smallpox expenditures will continue to dominate SNS spending.

The budget outlook also reveals a potential for a minimal emphasis in the coming years on basic smallpox or smallpox-relevant research at the National Institutes of Health (NIH) that would support the insertion of new drug candidates into the pipeline and a modest advanced development emphasis at the Biomedical Advanced Research and Development Agency (BARDA) for smallpox innovations. NIH is supporting the development of broadly protective monoclonal antibodies and mRNA-based vaccines for orthopoxviruses; BARDA is investing in a next-generation monoclonal antibody–based smallpox therapeutic. Citing lessons learned from COVID-19, the budget plan also relates "multidisciplinary" portfolios for BARDA and NIH that are designed to develop tools and platforms that cut across the CBRN space. PHEMCE expects a significantly increased need for funding in these multidisciplinary efforts, far outstripping any individual pathogen-specific budgetary line. The committee is interested to see how the predicted $16.5 billion over 5 years of investment (if funded) will support vaccine platforms, broad-spectrum therapeutics, and more rapid manufacturing options and the ways that such activities could benefit the smallpox portfolio.

The multi-year budget goes on to describe the smallpox MCM portfolio as "relatively more mature" in that it has reached a stage where costs are driven by sustainment and "investments in replenishment" rather than new investments (HHS, 2023). That is, the SNS is anticipating spending to primarily maintain a holding pattern regarding smallpox readiness. The description of BARDA's investment in smallpox MCMs includes funding to support sustained investment in a lyophilized formulation of MVA-BN, manufacturing of additional doses of MVA-BN to bolster domestic supply, and procurement of oral and intravenous tecovirimat to replenish products used to respond to the mpox outbreak. Sustainment of stockpiled assets is a prudent course, given the years and billions of dollars that have gone into developing and procuring these assets. Indeed, the lapse in BARDA's sustainment of stockpiled MVA-BN made national headlines when an outbreak forced the lapse—and its real-world impacts—into the light of day (Goldstein, 2022). These assets should not be developed only to be discarded.

And yet, the stockpile may be at an inflection point. With the SNS now more than two decades old, it stands to reason that some of its assets will have stood the test of time more than others. Ciprofloxacin and doxycycline are held to support anthrax response, and until BARDA's investments in antibacterial innovations begin to produce benefits, these antibiotics should be sustained. For smallpox, the scientific and technological opportunity for innovative and improved vaccines, therapeutics, and diagnostics may be a good argument for a transitional phase in which investments made to date are sustained to ensure a ready stockpile, while building a smallpox MCM stockpile of the future.

International Sharing of Burden and Benefit

The ongoing research and development of smallpox and orthopoxvirus MCMs need not be an enterprise taken on by the U.S. government alone. Collaborations and partnerships with other nations and organizations could offer platforms that would at once create a shared burden and enable a pathway toward international sharing of benefits.

Regional and global organizations are being founded to provide a pathway toward innovation and toward securing a regional or global supply of MCMs that can benefit populations beyond those that exist within national boundaries. The European Commission's 2021 Health Emergency Preparedness and Response Authority, or HERA, is designed to address market challenges in MCM readiness while fostering the international cooperation that will ensure availability and accessibility of those countermeasures globally (European Commission, n.d.). In 2022, Japan established the Strategic Center of Biomedical Advanced Vaccine Research and Development for Preparedness and Response, or SCARDA, to support commercialization of vaccines during non-pandemic settings with a view to achieving the G7 100 Days Mission for pandemic response (AMED, n.d.). The Coalition for Epidemic Preparedness, or CEPI, was established prior to the COVID-19 pandemic to accelerate MCM development for epidemic and pandemic threats and is a major player in 100-day efforts (CEPI, 2024). Philanthropies and governments invest in CEPI to support MCM research and development for pathogens from a number of viral families. CEPI has demonstrated success in developing partnerships and targeting investments to make new vaccines and make them accessible and affordable. For example, CEPI partnered with the EU's Horizon 2020 program in 2019 to invest $24.6 million in the first vaccine against chikungunya, IXCHIQ. CEPI's funding is devoted toward efforts to make IXCHIQ accessible to countries with the highest burden of disease, and not just available to travelers from high-income countries as originally anticipated (CEPI, 2023)

Such funders are well situated to support the development of next-generation smallpox and orthopoxvirus MCMs, and even to expand the use of those currently available. How the global community can most effectively build and leverage such organizations to support MCM innovation, development, stockpiling, and equitable dissemination remains under discussion. While the details lie outside the scope of this report, the committee emphasizes that the use of such structures could reduce the burden on the U.S. government alone to fund smallpox and orthopoxvirus MCMs.

Lessons From Mpox MCM SNS Deployment

BARDA investment in the advanced development of MCMs and SNS procurement of these and other assets, dating to the Project BioShield Act of 2004[2] have resulted in the nation being better protected against public health emergencies. Nevertheless, there is room for improvement.

The 2022 mpox outbreak may hold specific relevance to SNS considerations. The U.S. mpox response relied upon deploying stockpiled vaccines and antivirals, as would be the case for smallpox. MVA-BN was stockpiled for smallpox preparedness but had been approved by FDA for both smallpox and mpox (Adams, 2023; Wolfe, 2023). This reality meant that it became the go-to option for controlling the further spread of the mpox virus in the United States. An important question raised from the mpox experience is whether the dual indications for both a national security threat and an emerging infectious disease will remain an outlier, or whether it can

---

[2] Public Law: *Project BioShield Act of 2004*, Public Law 108-276, 108th Cong., 2d. sess. (July 21, 2004), 15.

and should be replicated. Such dual indications can meet BARDA's stated strategy to pursue solutions to emerging infectious disease that that can be adapted to and applied against a range threats (BARDA, 2022).

Unlike ACAM2000, the smallpox vaccine intended for the general population and thus stored in the large quantities, MVA-BN was intended for use in a subset of the population. So it was intentionally stockpiled in smaller amounts (Wolfe, 2023). This strained the response to mpox, which was not the pathogen for which it had been stockpiled. But critically, BARDA had let most of the millions of its finished SNS doses expire in favor of purchasing raw vaccine product to be held by the manufacturer internationally, dramatically affecting response time (Goldstein, 2022). This constrained the mpox response and would have also constrained a smallpox response.

Sufficient vaccine doses to support the population in need for mpox response were initially unavailable to meet demand. ASPR proceeded to order 5.5 million vials from the federal government's bulk supply held by Bavarian Nordic to be filled and finished, bringing the SNS supply to about 7 million vials by the middle of 2023; ASPR ultimately released more than 1 million single-use vials of MVA-BN to jurisdictions (ASPR, n.d.). ASPR also released stockpiled tecovirimat, and CDC worked on ensuring the availability of laboratory diagnostics for orthopoxviruses within the Laboratory Research Network and in commercial testing facilities (Aden et al., 2022; ASPR, n.d.).

Thus, the successes of the mpox response were tempered by major challenges, especially the short supply of immediately available vaccine doses, as well as by concerns over changes to dosing strategy during outbreak response, inequitable vaccine access, access to laboratory testing for patients, and overall federal, state, and local coordination (McQuiston, 2023; Mrsny, 2022).

It is important to learn from mpox while acknowledging and planning for the ways that a smallpox response would be different. The smallpox response plan assumes a full and fast mobilization (within 8 hours), or "push," of vaccine assets to pre-identified "ship to" locations, whereas the use of such a strategy was not used for mpox (Adams, 2023). Therapeutic options would be delivered upon request (pull) and shipped separately to points of care. Adams (2023) noted that the response strategy would be determined at time of incident collectively by federal and state, local, tribal, and territorial health officials. Furthermore, SNS officials noted to the committee that mpox presented as a threat localized to a particular demographic and required nationwide outreach and access targeted to this demographic.

While it is important to derive lessons from mpox outbreaks and SNS use, COVID-19 also provides many lessons, as described in prior chapters of this report. The constraints of CDC centrally managed diagnostics, a lack of research and development investment in rapid diagnostic technology in the years leading up to the outbreak, struggles with rapid vaccine manufacturing at scale, a dearth of therapeutics and inaccessibility of those treatments, and many other challenges provide a basis from which to make different decisions for smallpox preparedness.

Considerations for the Smallpox MCM Portfolio

The overall composition of the SNS has changed in the more than two decades since its inception (Kuiken and Gottron, 2023). It is not a static entity; its contents and concept of operations must evolve to meet evolving threats and to keep up with scientific and technological progress. These updates and changes are driven by the multi-step development process for the SNS annual review, including gap analyses and prioritizations, threat assessments (identifying new threats and revising existing threats), specific response scenarios, and by pharmaceutical advancements (GAO, 2022; Neumeister and Gray, 2021). The reality is that the time and expense required to research, develop, and approve new MCMs limits the ability to rapidly modify the SNS, but so too do entrenched ways of thinking about stockpiling strategies.

Over time, the SNS's role, responsibilities, and operational activities, and those of the MCM enterprise in general, have continued to significantly expand, sometimes without concomitant increases in resources (Kuiken and Gottron, 2023). The SNS is challenged with addressing many potential threats (expanding from chemical, biological, radiological, and nuclear (CBRN) to all-hazards and emerging infectious diseases) but in a resource-constrained environment that requires making prioritization decisions, or in some cases, decisions as if there were no costs involved at all (GAO, 2022). These decisions have strained the resources of the SNS and PHEMCE partners. However, many aspects of these challenges, such as defining the roles of the federal stockpile versus state or local stockpiles (an issue highlighted by recent experiences with COVID-19 and mpox), are beyond the scope of this report but deserve further examination. Similarly, new production technologies could dramatically affect how the SNS operates and what types of materials make sense for stockpiling (e.g., stockpiling of raw materials might be efficient if manufacturing agreements are in place and platform technologies are developed that can rapidly produce a variety of different vaccines—or diagnostics or therapeutics—from the same materials). The committee believes that these platform technologies are worth pursuing and as mentioned in Chapter 3 the new Biopharmaceutical Manufacturing Preparedness Consortium could play a role in bringing new technologies to bear, but until they are proven successful, the SNS will need to continue to stockpile MCMs (GAO, 2023).

Project BioShield was designed to support the acquisition by the SNS of countermeasures under development for national security threats (Kuiken and Gottron, 2023). BARDA's remit based upon this law has been to support the stockpiling of MCMs for CBRN threats. In general, MCMs for CBRN threats lack a commercial market and in some cases are explicitly disallowed from being sold to any entity other than the federal government. For smallpox-specific countermeasures, the federal government (and other governments internationally) have been the only buyers. State, local, tribal, or territorial governments are not required to maintain their own stockpiles of medical and ancillary equipment to prepare for and respond to any public health emergency, including smallpox (Kuiken and Gottron, 2023). The experience with mpox, however, may necessitate a change in the way smallpox readiness is viewed, in the sense that a growing need for commercially available mpox countermeasures could incentivize innovation and investment in MCMs that also support the federal government–centric responsibility for smallpox MCM preparedness.

To aid SNS administrators in their review of the future of the SNS smallpox MCM portfolio, the committee poses the following considerations (Box 4-2). The SNS may be the purchaser of available MCM and needed supplies, but BARDA is responsible for the advanced development that makes products possible, and members of the PHEMCE contribute to early development, regulatory, and other elements of the chain of investments and decisions that make SNS assets possible (NASEM, 2021). BARDA currently develops target product profiles (TPPs) for specific MCMs (BARDA, n.d.; FIND, n.d.; IOM, 2010; NIAID, 2023). TPPs can help guide industry, regulatory agencies, procurers, and funders on research and development priorities. To inform their future priorities for the smallpox MCM portfolio, BARDA and PHEMCE could develop new TPPs and refine existing TPPs for smallpox MCMs. This could include defining the product, including both the indication (i.e., disease/condition to be treated) and what an appropriate product would be to use in a public health emergency, prospectively establishing the metrics that define success for a product, and then building an experimental plan that assesses whether a product has critical attributes. Currently, BARDA has a TPP for smallpox vaccine, which could be refined and updated, and TPPs could be created for smallpox therapeutics and diagnostics. WHO also developed two diagnostic TPPs during the global mpox response and recommended that TPPs be developed for smallpox diagnostics (WHO, 2022b, 2023).

BOX 4-2
Considerations for and Questions About
Smallpox MCMs in the SNS

High-Level Assessment

- *Articulating different goals and milestones depending on MCM portfolio maturity.* The smallpox MCM portfolio is a mature portfolio, and the goals of the portfolio should differ from a relatively new MCM portfolio.
- *Examine the potential uses of and implications for currently stockpiled MCMs for other orthopoxvirus outbreaks.* Consider the threat of other orthopoxviruses that stockpiled smallpox MCMs could be used for, and furthermore, if mpox becomes a more serious global health problem, consider the risk of further depletion of stockpiled smallpox MCMs.
- *Diversifying stockpiled smallpox MCMs.* The development and stockpiling of multiple MCMs may mitigate the risk of supply shortages and address potential efficacy, safety, pricing, administration, and uptake concerns, but it may also amplify sustainability concerns absent a commercial market for the products.
- *Developing a framework to guide decision making if new smallpox MCMs are developed.* For example, there is the possibility that assets for non-variola orthopoxviruses could appear on the market through private investment or the investment of other governments. The SNS will need a basis for considering whether and how these could support progress toward smallpox preparedness.
- *Optimizing maintenance and sustainment of current smallpox MCM stockpile.* As the SNS has shifted toward primarily sustaining the smallpox MCM stockpile, consider efforts and technology to reduce the cost of sustainment. For example, ongoing trials on freeze-dried formulation of MVA-BN could also present improved storage options for this vaccine compared with liquid formulation.
- *Re-evaluating assumptions.* Stockpiling assumptions may need to consider the possibility of an increase or reduction in effective doses after potency testing against the disease-causing strain in an actual smallpox event. Similarly, ring vaccination or other vaccination strategies, vaccine hesitancy, and/or the existence of effective therapeutics might alter assumptions of a vaccine stockpile.
- *Planning for loss of manufacturing capacity.* Because the SNS relies on just a few manufacturers for smallpox MCMs, it is important to assess how a loss of manufacturing capacity from any given company could affect readiness and response and could inform strategies to ensure stability of the manufacturing base.

Operationalization: Rapid Deployment

- *Reviewing the deployment-ready stockpile formulation.* To ensure smallpox MCMs are ready to be deployed as quickly as possible.
- *Updating response plans and training and exercise tools to reflect current and potential new smallpox MCMs.* Consider issues such as multiple outbreak scenarios, triggers, and the scope of the required response (scalable plans and surge capacity). For example, plans may need to include how existing stockpiled vaccines would be used in the classic ring vaccination strategy or other vaccination strategies, and the number of doses needed, based on transmission of three to six new cases (reproductive number) from each case. Similarly, plans for the deployment of treatments based on exercised scenarios could further assist in defining short-term and longer-term needs during the emergency.

continued

BOX 4-2 Continued

- *Planning for implementation, coordination, and communication considerations up front.* This may include research and development on topics such as logistics, equitable access and distribution of smallpox MCMs (e.g., allocation frameworks, transparent decision-making processes), information sharing, risk communication, and education and training for frontline responders.

MCM-Specific Stockpiling Considerations and Questions

- *Understanding the specific indications and requirements of each MCM* (e.g., supply sources/challenges; delivery needs; handling and storage requirements; shelf life and shelf-life extension, vendor-managed inventory, and optimal timing of administration for greatest efficacy; and adverse effects).
- Vaccines
  - How often titer is checked on existing lots held by the SNS, in what form are they stored (e.g., lyophilized and refrigerated or frozen and at what temperature versus liquid frozen and at what temperature), and how often are the lots checked for titer and loss of same and the titer loss curves examined?
  - What is the appropriate mix of single-use vials, multidose vials, or pre-filled syringes?
  - What is the appropriate mix of frozen versus lyophilized?
  - Could the stockpiling strategy change to stockpile starter volumes of virus for vaccines?
  - Should sustaining stores of smallpox vaccines be viewed as an irrevocable obligation while purchases of other products for the SNS are discretionary? And what is a reasonable price to pay for new vaccine doses to replace expiring doses?
- Therapeutics
  - What is the estimated minimal initial need, based on simulation exercises for smallpox as well as mpox?
  - Is there any repurposing of the therapeutic that would permit commercialization of the therapeutic agent and thereby reduce the needed size of the stockpile?
  - How long will it take to manufacture more of each needed therapeutic agents?
- Diagnostics
  - Should the SNS include specimen collection supplies?
  - How are federal and state testing strategies for variola in an outbreak different from what was used during mpox (e.g., differences in biosafety designation, higher marginal cost of a false positive, and unique epidemiology), and how does this affect downstream choices in terms of test deployment and placement as well as specimen transportation?

Conclusions on the SNS and Smallpox MCM Portfolio

(4-4) The nation relies on the SNS to deploy MCMs in response to a smallpox event because, currently, most of the necessary MCMs are not commercially available. Moving forward, leveraging collaborations and partnerships with other nations and organizations to develop next-generation smallpox and orthopoxvirus MCMs and expanding the use of the current ones could create a shared burden and enable a pathway toward international sharing of benefits.

(4-5) To facilitate a successful response in the event of a smallpox outbreak, the suite of smallpox MCMs (diagnostics, vaccines, and therapeutics) will be deployed and must work in concert with one another. However, the smallpox MCM suite has not been tested or exercised in this way: These MCMs were not used during the smallpox eradication campaign, some have not been deployed simultaneously before, and some are based on older technology and use outdated assumptions, including changes in population (e.g., demographic, physiological, and behavioral/risk perception).

(4-6) Threat assessments and specific response scenarios, based on different potential smallpox or orthopoxvirus events, are needed to assess and determine the necessary quantities and types of MCMs needed for various effective and equitable response strategies (e.g., early detection, immediate versus long-term response, isolation of patients, quarantine of contacts, use of therapeutics for prophylaxis and treatment including pre-exposure prophylaxis with therapeutics for first responders and health care providers, ring vaccination, or mass vaccination).

OVERARCHING CONCLUSIONS

Despite the research done over recent decades and the fact that there are more smallpox MCMs available now than there were in the pre-eradication period, the nation's readiness and response posture to a smallpox outbreak could be strengthened. Based on the evidence and findings on the utility of live variola virus for research and the smallpox MCM portfolio planning, the committee drew the following overarching conclusions:

For the foreseeable future, some research with live variola virus remains essential to achieving public health research goals against an ever-evolving biothreat landscape and the potential for orthopoxviruses to emerge naturally or deliberately.

The smallpox MCM portfolio is a mature portfolio, and the goals of a mature portfolio should differ from a relatively new MCM portfolio. The scientific and technological opportunity for innovative and improved smallpox MCMs supports a transitional phase for the smallpox MCM portfolio, in which investments made to date are sustained to ensure a ready stockpile—while leveraging collaborations and partnerships with other nations and organizations to build a diversified smallpox MCM stockpile and an agile, on-demand, distributed MCM response network of the future.

REFERENCES

Adams, S. A. 2023. Strategic National Stockpile smallpox medical countermeasures overview. Presentation at Meeting 3 of the Committee on Current State of Research, Development, and Stockpiling of Smallpox MCMs of the National Academies. December 14. https://www.nationalacademies. org/event/41411_12-2023_meeting-3-of-the-committee-on-the-current-state-of-research-development-and-stockpiling-of-smallpox-medical-countermeasures (accessed February 18, 2024).

Aden, T. A., P. Blevins, S. W. York, S. Rager, D. Balachandran, C. L. Hutson, D. Lowe, C. N. Mangal, T. Wolford, and A. Matheny. 2022. Rapid diagnostic testing for response to the monkeypox outbreak—Laboratory Response Network, United States, May 17–June 30, 2022. *Morbidity and Mortality Weekly Report* 71(28):904.

Altindis, M., E. Puca, and L. Shapo. 2022. Diagnosis of monkeypox virus—An overview. *Travel Medicine and Infectious Disease* 50:102459.

AMED (Japan Agency for Medical Research and Development). n.d. *Strategic Center of Biomedical Advanced Vaccine Research and Development for Preparedness and Response.* https://www.amed. go.jp/en/program/list/21/index.html (accessed February 27, 2024).

ASPR (Administration for Strategic Preparedness and Response). n.d. *Response to the Mpox outbreak: Strategic National Stockpile.* https://aspr.hhs.gov/SNS/Pages/Response-to-Monkeypox.aspx (accessed January 15, 2024).

BARDA (Biomedical Advanced Research and Development Authority). 2022. *BARDA strategic plan (2022–2026).* https://medicalcountermeasures.gov/media/38717/barda-strategic-plan-2022-2026.pdf (accessed February 29, 2024).

BARDA. n.d. *Barda target profiles.* https://medicalcountermeasures.gov/barda/tpp (accessed February 6, 2024).

CEPI (Coalition for Epidemic Preparedness Innovations). 2023. *Accelerating access to the world's first Chikungunya vaccine.* https://cepi.net/news_cepi/accelerating-access-to-the-worlds-first-chikungunya-vaccine (acccessed February 27, 2024).

CEPI. 2024. Preparing for future pandemics. https://cepi.net (accessed February 27, 2024).

Damaso, C. R., J. J. Esposito, R. C. Condit, and N. Moussatché. 2000. An emergent poxvirus from humans and cattle in Rio de Janeiro State: Cantagalo virus may derive from Brazilian smallpox vaccine. *Virology* 277(2):439–449.

Damon, I. K., C. R. Damaso, and G. McFadden. 2014. Are we there yet? The smallpox research agenda using variola virus. *PLOS Pathogens* 10(5):e1004108.

Deng, L., P. Dai, A. Ciro, D. F. Smee, H. Djaballah, and S. Shuman. 2007. Identification of novel antipoxviral agents: Mitoxantrone inhibits vaccinia virus replication by blocking virion assembly. *Journal of Virology* 81(24):13392–13402.

Dower, K., C. M. Filone, E. N. Hodges, Z. B. Bjornson, K. H. Rubins, L. E. Brown, S. Schaus, L. E. Hensley, and J. H. Connor. 2012. Identification of a pyridopyrimidinone inhibitor of orthopoxviruses from a diversity-oriented synthesis library. *Journal of Virology* 86(5):2632–2640.

European Commission. n.d. *Health Emergency Preparedness and Response (HERA).* https://health. ec.europa.eu/health-emergency-preparedness-and-response-hera_en (accessed February 27, 2024).

Fang, Z., V. S. Monteiro, P. A. Renauer, X. Shang, K. Suzuki, X. Ling, M. Bai, Y. Xiang, A. Levchenko, C. J. Booth, C. Lucas, and S. Chen. 2023. Polyvalent mRNA vaccination elicited potent immune response to monkeypox virus surface antigens. *Cell Research* 33(5):407–410.

FDA (U.S. Food and Drug Administration). 2018. *510(k) substantial equivalence determination decision summary (K181205).* https://www.accessdata.fda.gov/cdrh_docs/reviews/K181205.pdf (accessed February 18, 2024).

FDA. n.d. Monkeypox fast facts: TPOXX (tecovirimat). https://www.fda.gov/media/160480/download (accessed February 18, 2024).

FIND. n.d. *Target product profiles.* https://www.finddx.org/tools-and-resources/rd-and-innovation/ target-product-profiles (accessed February 6, 2024).

Freyn, A. W., C. Atyeo, P. L. Earl, J. L. Americo, G. Y. Chuang, H. Natarajan, T. R. Frey, J. G. Gall, J. I. Moliva, R. Hunegnaw, G. Asthagiri Arunkumar, C. O. Ogega, A. Nasir, G. Santos, R. H. Levin, A. Meni, P. A. Jorquera, H. Bennett, J. A. Johnson, M. A. Durney, G. Stewart-Jones, J. W. Hooper, T. M. Colpitts, G. Alter, N. J. Sullivan, A. Carfi, and B. Moss. 2023. An mpox virus mRNA–lipid nanoparticle vaccine confers protection against lethal orthopoxviral challenge. *Science Translational Medicine* 15(716):eadg3540.

GAO (Government Accountability Office). 2022. *Public Health Preparedness: HHS Should Address Strategic National Stockpile Requirements and Inventory Risks (GAO-23-106210)*. Washington, DC: Government Accountability Office.

GAO. 2023. *Public health preparedness: HHS should plan for medical countermeasure development and manufacturing risks (GAO-23-105713)*. Washington, DC: Government Accountability Office.

Goldstein, J. 2022. How the U.S. let 20 million doses of monkeypox vaccine expire. *The New York Times*, August 1.

Griffin, D. O., D. Brennan-Rieder, B. Ngo, P. Kory, M. Confalonieri, L. Shapiro, J. Iglesias, M. Dube, N. Nanda, G. K. In, D. Arkfeld, P. Chaudhary, V. M. Campese, D. L. Hanna, D. Sawcer, G. Ehresmann, D. Peng, M. Smorgorzewski, A. Amstrong, E. H. Vinjevoll, R Dasgupta, F. R. Sattler, C. Mussini, O. Mitja, V. Soriano, N. Peschanski, G. Hayem, M. C. Piccirillo, A. Lobo-Ferreira, I. B. Rivero, I. F. H. Hung, M. Rendell, S. Ditmore, J. Varon, and P. Marik. 2021. The importance of understanding the states of COVID-19 in treatment and trials. *AIDS Reviews* 23(1):40–47.

Hedberg, H., and A. Zink. 2024. *Fatal Alaskapox infection in a Southcentral Alaska resident*. State of Alaska Epidemiology Bulletin. https://epi.alaska.gov/bulletins/docs/b2024_02.pdf (accessed February 15, 2024).

HHS (Department of Health and Human Services). 2023. *Public Health Emergency Medical Countermeasures Enterprise multiyear budget: Fiscal years 2022–2026*. https://aspr.hhs.gov/PHEMCE/Documents/2022-2026-PHEMCE-Budget.pdf (accessed February 18, 2024).

Hooper, J. W., D. M. Custer, and E. Thompson. 2003. Four-gene-combination DNA vaccine protects mice against a lethal vaccinia virus challenge and elicits appropriate antibody responses in non-human primates. *Virology* 306(1):181–195.

Hou, F., Y. Zhang, X. Liu, Y. M. Murad, J. Xu, Z. Yu, X. Hua, Y. Song, J. Ding, H. Huang, R. Zhao, W. Jia, and X. Yang. 2023. mRNA vaccines encoding fusion proteins of monkeypox virus antigens protect mice from vaccinia virus challenge. *Nature Communications* 14(1):5925.

Huggins, J., A. Goff, L. Hensley, E. Mucker, J. Shamblin, C. Wlazlowski, W. Johnson, J. Chapman, T. Larsen, N. Twenhafel, K. Karem, I. K. Damon, C. M. Byrd, T. C. Bolken, R. Jordan, and D. Hruby. 2009. Nonhuman primates are protected from smallpox virus or monkeypox virus challenges by the antiviral drug ST-246. *Antimicrobial Agents and Chemotherapy* 53(6):2620–2625.

Hutson, C. 2023. Variola virus research—Overview of main activities and use of live virus. Presentation at Meeting 2 of the Committee on Current State of Research, Development, and Stockpiling of Smallpox MCMs. December 1. https://www.nationalacademies.org/event/41410_12-2023_meeting-2-of-the-committee-on-the-current-state-of-research-development-and-stockpiling-of-smallpox-medical-countermeasures (accessed February 18, 2024).

Hutson, C. L., A. V. Kondas, J. M. Ritter, Z. Reed, S. D. Ostergaard, C. N. Morgan, N. Gallardo-Romero, C. Tansey, M. R. Mauldin, J. S. Salzer, C. M. Hughes, C. S. Goldsmith, D. Carroll, and V. A. Olson. 2021. Teaching a new mouse old tricks: Humanized mice as an infection model for variola virus. *PLOS Pathogens* 17(9):e1009633.

IOM (Institute of Medicine). 1999. *Assessment of future scientific needs for live variola virus*. Washington, DC: National Academy Press.

IOM. 2009. *Live variola virus: Considerations for continuing research*. Washington, DC: The National Academies Press.

IOM. 2010. *The Public Health Emergency Medical Countermeasures Enterprise: Innovative strategies to enhance products from discovery through approval: Workshop summary*. Washington, DC: The National Academies Press.

Kuiken, T., and F. Gottron. 2023. *The Strategic National Stockpile: Overview and issues for Congress.* Congressional Research Services R47400. https://crsreports.congress.gov/product/pdf/R/R47400 (accessed February 18, 2024).

Lewis, R. 2023. Variola virus research—Overview of main activities and use of live virus. Presentation at Meeting 2 of the Committee on Current State of Research, Development, and Stockpiling of Smallpox MCMs. December 1. https://www.nationalacademies.org/event/41410_12-2023_meeting-2-of-the-committee-on-the-current-state-of-research-development-and-stockpiling-of-smallpox-medical-countermeasures (accessed February 18, 2024).

Li, Y., V. A. Olson, T. Laue, M. T. Laker, and I. K. Damon. 2006. Detection of monkeypox virus with real-time PCR assays. *Journal of Clinical Virology* 36(3):194–203.

Linas, B. P., and C. O. Cunningham. 2019. Coronavirus disease 2019 (COVID-19) disparities: A call for equity in health outcomes and clinical research. *Clinical Infectious Diseases* 73(11):e4139–e4140.

Low, S. J., M. T. O'Neill, W. J. Kerry, M. Krysiak, G. Papadakis, L. W. Whitehead, I. Savic, J. Prestedge, L. Williams, J. P. Cooney, T. Tran, C. K. Lim, L. Caly, J. M. Towns, C. S. Bradshaw, C. Fairley, E. P. F. Chow, M. Y. Chen, M. Pellegrini, S. Pasricha, and D. A. Williamson. 2023. Rapid detection of monkeypox virus using a CRISPR-Cas12a mediated assay: A laboratory validation and evaluation study. *The Lancet Microbe* 4(10):e800–e810.

McQuiston, J. H. 2023. The CDC domestic mpox response—United States, 2022–2023.*Morbidity and Mortality Weekly Report* 72(20):547–552.

Moss, B., and G. L. Smith. 2021. Chapter 16: *Poxviridae*: The viruses and their replication. In P. M. Howley and D. M. Knipe (eds.), *Fields virology: DNA viruses, vol. 2 (7th edition).* Philadelphia: Wolters Kluwer Health. Pp. 573–613.

Mrsny, R. J., 2022. Does an intradermal vaccination for monkeypox make sense? *The AAPS Journal* 24(6):104.

Mulangu, S., L. E. Dodd, R. T. Davey Jr., O. T. Mbaya, M. Proschan, D. Mukadi, M. L. Manzo, D. Nzolo, A. T. Oloma, A. Ibanda, R. Ali, S. Coulibaly, A. C. Levine, R. Grais, J. Diaz, H. C. Lane, J. Muyembe-Tamfum, PALM Writing Group, B. Sivahera, M. Camara, R. Kojan, R. Walker, B. Dighero-Kemp, H. Cao, P. Mukumbayi, P. Mbala-Kingebeni, S. Ahuka, S. Albert, T. Bonnett, I. Crozier, M. Duvenhage, C. Proffitt, M. Teitelbaum, T. Moench, J. Aboulhab, K. Barrett, K. Cahill, K. Cone, R. Eckes, L. Hensley, B. Herpin, E. Higgs, J. Ledgerwood, J. Pierson, M. Smolskis, Y. Sow, J. Tierney, S. Sivapalasingam, W. Holman, N. Gettinger, D. Vallee, J. Nordwall, and PALM Consortium Study Team. 2019. A randomized, controlled trial of Ebola virus disease therapeutics. *New England Journal of Medicine* 381(24):2293–2303.

NASEM (National Academies of Sciences, Engineering, and Medicine). 2017. *Integrating clinical research into epidemic response: The Ebola experience.* Washington, DC: The National Academies Press.

NASEM. 2021. *Ensuring an effective public health emergency medical countermeasures enterprise.* Washington, DC: The National Academies Press.

Neumeister, S. M., and J. P. Gray. 2021. The Strategic National Stockpile: Identification, support, and acquisition of medical countermeasures for CBRN incidents. *Toxicology Mechanisms and Methods* 31(4):308–321.

NIAID (National Institute of Allergy and Infectious Diseases). 2023. *Target product profiles for antivirals.* https://www.niaid.nih.gov/research/target-product-profiles-antivirals (accessed February 6, 2024).

Olson, V. A., S. K. Smith, S. Foster, Y. Li, E. R. Lanier, I. Gates, L. C. Trost, and I. K. Damon. 2014. In vitro efficacy of brincidofovir against variola virus. *Antimicrobial Agents and Chemotherapy* 58(9):5570–5571.

Peng, C., Y. Zhou, S. Cao, A. Pant, M. L. Campos Guerrero, P. McDonald, A. Roy, and Z. Yang. 2020. Identification of vaccinia virus inhibitors and cellular functions necessary for efficient viral replication by screening bioactives and FDA-approved drugs. *Vaccines* 8(3):401.

Petrini, C., C. Mannelli, L. Riva, S. Gainotti, and G. Gussoni. 2022. Decentralized clinical trials (DCTs): A few ethical considerations. *Frontiers in Public Health* 10:1081150.

Rcheulishvili, N., J. Mao, D. Papukashvili, S. Feng, C. Liu, X. Yang, J. Lin, Y. He, and P. G. Wang. 2023. Development of a multi-epitope universal mRNA vaccine candidate for monkeypox, smallpox, and vaccinia viruses: Design and in silico analyses. *Viruses* 15(5):1120.

Robinson, P. C., D. F. L. Liew, H. L. Tanner, J. R. Grainger, R. A. Dwek, R. B. Reisler, L. Steinman, M. Feldmann, L. P. Ho, T. Hussell, P. Moss, D. Richards, and N. Zitzmann. 2022. COVID-19 therapeutics: Challenges and directions for the future. *Proceedings of the National Academy of Sciences* 119(15):e2119893119.

Russo, A. T., D. W. Grosenbach, J. Chinsangaram, K. M. Honeychurch, P. G. Long, C. Lovejoy, B. Maiti, I. Meara, and D. E. Hruby. 2021. An overview of tecovirimat for smallpox treatment and expanded anti-orthopoxvirus applications. *Expert Review of Anti-Infective Therapy* 19(3):331–344. https://doi.org/10.1080/14787210.2020.1819791.

Sang, Y., Z. Zhang, F. Liu, H. Lu, C. Yu, H. Sun, J. Long, Y. Cao, J. Mai, Y. Miao, X. Wang, J. Fang, Y. Wang, W. Huang, J. Yang, and S. Wang. 2023. Monkeypox virus quadrivalent mRNA vaccine induces immune response and protects against vaccinia virus. *Signal Transduction and Targeted Therapy* 8(1):172.

Satheshkumar, P. S., and I. K. Damon. 2021. Chapter 17: Poxviruses. In P. M. Howley and D. M. Knipe (eds.), *Fields virology: DNA viruses, vol. 2 (7th edition)*. Philadelphia: Wolters Kluwer. Pp. 614–640.

Stabenow, J., R. M. Buller, J. Schriewer, C. West, J. E. Sagartz, and S. Parker. 2010. A mouse model of lethal infection for evaluating prophylactics and therapeutics against monkeypox virus. *Journal of Virology* 84(8):3909–3920.

Stefano, J. S., L. R. G. e Silva, C. Kalinke, P. R. de Oliveira, R. D. Crapnell, L. C. Brazaca, J. A. Bonacin, S. Campuzano, C. E. Banks, and B. C. Janegitz. 2023. Human monkeypox virus: Detection methods and perspectives for diagnostics. *TrAC Trends in Analytical Chemistry* 167:117226.

White House. 2022. *National biodefense strategy and implementation plan for countering biological threats, enhancing pandemic preparedness, and achieving global health security, October 2022.* https://www.whitehouse.gov/wp-content/uploads/2022/10/National-Biodefense-Strategy-and-Implementation-Plan-Final.pdf (accessed February 18, 2024).

WHO (World Health Organization). 2010. *Advisory Group of Independent Experts to review the smallpox research programme (AGIES): Comments on the scientific review of variola virus research, 1999–2010.* Geneva: World Health Organization. https://www.who.int/publications/i/item/WHO-HSE-GAR-BDP-2010-4 (accessed February 18, 2024).

WHO. 2013. *Advisory Group of Independent Experts to review the smallpox research programme (AGIES): Report to the World Health Organization.* Geneva: World Health Organization. https://www.who.int/publications/i/item/WHO-HSE-PED-CED-2013-3 (accessed February 18. 2024).

WHO. 2022a. *Strengthening clinical trials to provide high-quality evidence on health interventions and to improve research quality and coordination.* https://apps.who.int/gb/ebwha/pdf_files/WHA75/A75_R8-en.pdf (accessed February 18, 2024).

WHO. 2022b. *WHO target product profile (TPP) therapeutics for monkeypox cases* https://cdn.who.int/media/docs/default-source/blue-print/who_monkeypox_therapeutic_draft-tpp_august-2022.pdf (accessed February 6, 2024).

WHO. 2023. *WHO Advisory Committee on Variola Virus Research: Report of the twenty-fourth meeting, Geneva, 29–30 November 2022.* https://www.who.int/publications/i/item/9789240076310 (accessed February 18, 2024).

WHO. 2024a. *154th session of the executive board, provisional agenda item 18 —Smallpox eradication: Destruction of variola virus stocks (January 2, 2024).* https://apps.who.int/gb/ebwha/pdf_files/EB154/B154_20-en.pdf (accessed February 18, 2024).

WHO. 2024b. *Advisory Committee for Variola Virus Research: About us.* https://www.who.int/groups/who-advisory-committee-on-variola-virus-research/about (accessed February 1, 2024).

WHO. n.d. *Research using live variola virus.* https://www.who.int/activities/research-using-live-variola-virus (accessed February 4, 2024).

Wolfe, D. 2023. Smallpox vaccines overview. Presentation at Meeting 3 of the Committee on Current State of Research, Development, and Stockpiling of Smallpox MCMs of the National Academies. December 14. https://www.nationalacademies.org/event/41411_12-2023_meeting-3-of-the-committee-on-the-current-state-of-research-development-and-stockpiling-of-smallpox-medical-countermeasures (accessed February 23, 2024).

Yang, G., D. C. Pevear, M. H. Davies, M. S. Collett, T. Bailey, S. Rippen, L. Barone, C. Burns, G. Rhodes, S. Tohan, J. W. Huggins, R. O. Baker, R. L. Buller, E. Touchette, K. Waller, J. Schriewer, J. Neyts, E. DeClercq, K. Jones, D. Hruby, and R. Jordan. 2005. An orally bioavailable antipoxvirus compound (ST-246) inhibits extracellular virus formation and protects mice from lethal orthopoxvirus challenge. *Journal of Virology* 79(20):13139–13149.

Yang, X., C. Hu, X. Yang, X. Yang, X. Hu, X. Wang, C. Liu, Y. Yuan, S. Du, P. G. Wang, and J. Lin. 2023. Evaluation and comparison of immune responses induced by two mpox mRNA vaccine candidates in mice. *Journal of Medical Virology* 95(10):e29140.

Zeng, J., Y. Li, L. Jiang, L. Luo, Y. Wang, H. Wang, X. Han, J. Zhao, G. Gu, M. Fang, Q. Huang, and J. Yan. 2023. Mpox multi-antigen mRNA vaccine candidates by a simplified manufacturing strategy afford efficient protection against lethal orthopoxvirus challenge. *Emerging Microbes & Infections* 12(1):2204151.

Zhang, R. R., Z. J. Wang, Y. L. Zhu, W. Tang, C. Zhou, S. Q. Zhao, M. Wu, T. Ming, Y. Q. Deng, Q. Chen, N. Y. Jin, Q. Ye, X. Li, and C. F. Qin. 2023. Rational development of multicomponent mRNA vaccine candidates against mpox. *Emerging Microbes & Infections* 12(1):2192815.

Zimmer, C. 2021. How the search for COVID-19 treatments faltered while vaccines sped ahead. *The New York Times*, September 28.

A

Study Methods and Public Meeting Agendas

At the request of the Administration for Strategic Preparedness and Response (ASPR), the National Academies of Sciences, Engineering, and Medicine (the National Academies) convened the Committee on the Current State of Research, Development, and Stockpiling of Smallpox Medical Countermeasures. In addressing its charge and preparing its final report, the committee pursued several avenues for information collection and analysis. This appendix describes the committee's study process, including copies of the public meeting agendas.

MEETINGS AND INFORMATION-GATHERING ACTIVITIES

The committee held five virtual full committee meetings from November 2023 through February 2024. The committee held three meetings that included portions open to the public as well as one virtual public workshop. The agendas for these four open sessions are included at the end of this appendix.

To inform its deliberations, the committee gathered information through a variety of mechanisms including a review of literature from 2009 and were informed by reports and deliberations of the 154th session of the World Health Organization (WHO) Executive Board. Targeted literature reviews were conducted as novel issues arose throughout the committee's deliberations. All written information provided to the committee from external sources is available by request through the National Academies' Public Access Records Office.

PUBLIC AGENDAS

MEETING 1 AGENDA

Thursday, November 16, 2023

Purpose
- Hear from the sponsoring agency on their perspective of the statement of task and to hear from relevant stakeholders.
- Identify core issues to be addressed in the report.

OPEN SESSION

Sponsor Briefing: Discussion of the Committee's Charge

Objectives: *To hear from the sponsors of the study regarding their perspectives on the charge to the committee.*

2:00 p.m.	**Welcoming Remarks** LARRY GOSTIN, *Committee Chair* Distinguished University Professor and O'Neill Chair in Global Health Law O'Neill Institute for National and Global Health Law Georgetown University
2:05 p.m.	**Sponsor Perspective on Charge to the Committee** Administration for Strategic Preparedness and Response (ASPR)
3:30 p.m.	**ADJOURN**

MEETING 2 AGENDA

Friday, December 1, 2023

Purpose
- Hold an open session to hear from different U.S. government and international partners on key activities and perspectives relevant to the charge.
- Hear from subject matter experts on different issues related to variola and poxvirus research and medical countermeasure development.

OPEN SESSION

2:00 p.m.	**Welcoming Remarks** LARRY GOSTIN, *Committee Chair* Distinguished University Professor and O'Neill Chair in Global Health Law O'Neill Institute for National and Global Health Law Georgetown University
2:05 p.m.	**Variola Virus Research—Overview of Main Activities** **and Use of Live Virus** CHRISTY HUTSON Chief, Poxvirus and Rabies Branch Division of High Consequence Pathogens and Pathology U.S. Centers for Disease Control and Prevention (CDC) ROSAMUND LEWIS Head, WHO Smallpox Secretariat, Technical Lead for Orthopoxviruses World Health Organization (WHO)
3:15 p.m.	**Perspectives from Prominent Poxvirus Researchers** BERNARD MOSS Chief, Genetic Engineering Section National Institute of Allergy and Infectious Diseases (NIAID) STUART ISAACS Associate Professor of Medicine Perelman School of Medicine University of Pennsylvania
4:00 p.m.	**ADJOURN**

PUBLIC WORKSHOP AGENDA (DAY 1)

Thursday, December 14, 2023

Purpose
- Hold an open session to hear from different U.S. government partners on key activities relevant to the charge.
- Examine the current state of medical countermeasures (MCMs) for the diagnosis, prevention, and treatment of smallpox, including the continued role of live variola virus for research and public health purposes.
- Explore how lessons learned from COVID-19 and mpox can inform future preparedness and readiness.
- Examine potential scenarios and strategies that might inform future stockpiling of smallpox MCMs.

SESSION I Day 1 Opening Session

12:00 p.m.   **Welcoming Remarks**
LARRY GOSTIN, *Committee Chair*
Distinguished University Professor and O'Neill Chair in Global Health Law
O'Neill Institute for National and Global Health Law
Georgetown University

SESSION II U.S. Government Updates

Objectives: *Hear briefings from federal stakeholders on current activities for smallpox medical countermeasures.*

Guiding Questions:
- What is the current regulatory landscape for smallpox medical countermeasures?
- What is the current research and development landscape for smallpox medical countermeasures?
- What is the current state of stockpiling of smallpox medical countermeasures?
- What additional areas of research and development could be conducted to improve our MCMs?

NOREEN HYNES, *Moderator, Committee Member*

12:05 p.m.   **U.S. Food and Drug Administration Panel**
                  NOEL GERALD
                  Branch Chief for Bacterial Respiratory and Medical
                  Countermeasures
                  Division of Microbiology Devices, Center for Devices
                  and Radiological Health
                  FDA

12:20 p.m.   **Administration for Strategic Preparedness and
                  Response Panel**
                  STEVE ADAMS
                  Director, Strategic National Stockpile
                  ASPR

                  DANIEL WOLFE
                  Branch Chief, CBRN Vaccines
                  BARDA

                  KAREN MARTINS
                  Branch Chief, CBRN Antivirals and Antitoxins
                  BARDA

                  MARGARET SLOANE
                  Office of Strategy, Policy, and Requirements
                  ASPR

SESSION III Smallpox Medical Countermeasures Landscape

Objectives: *(1) Examine current state of MCMs for the prevention and treatment of smallpox, and (2) explore how lessons learned from COVID-19 and mpox can inform future preparedness and readiness.*

Guiding Questions:
- What is the current research and development landscape for smallpox medical countermeasures?
- How effective are the current MCMs for the diagnosis, prevention, and treatment of smallpox?
- What additional areas of research and development could be conducted to improve our MCMs?
- How did the mpox outbreak alter assumptions about the efficacy and utility of smallpox MCMs?
- How can the lessons from COVID-19 and mpox inform the U.S. preparedness and readiness posture?

2:05 p.m.   **Vaccine Research and Development**
                   RICK KENNEDY, *Moderator, Committee Member*

                   PAUL CHAPLIN
                   Chief Executive Officer
                   Bavarian Nordic

                   SETH LEDERMAN
                   Co-Founder, Chief Executive Officer, and Chairman
                   Tonix

                   BRETT LEAV
                   Head, Clinical Development, Public Health Vaccines
                   Moderna

                   CHRIS SINCLAIR
                   Head of Global Preparedness Government Business
                   Emergent BioSolutions

3:05 p.m.   **Therapeutics Research and Development**
                   INGER DAMON, *Moderator, Committee Member*

                   CYRUS JAVAN
                   Medical Officer
                   Division of AIDS
                   NIAID

                   DENNIS HRUBY
                   Chief Scientific Officer
                   SIGA

SESSION IV Scenario Planning and MCM Stockpiling Strategies

Objectives: *(1) Explore how recent COVID-19 and mpox public health emergencies have altered assumptions about the U.S. preparedness, readiness, and MCMs stockpiling posture for smallpox, and (2) examine potential scenarios and strategies that might inform future stockpiling of smallpox MCMs.*

Guiding Questions:
- How has the mpox outbreak altered our assumption about the availability of smallpox MCMs and the ability to meet potential global demand?
- How do advancements in biotechnology, life sciences research, and converging and enabling technologies alter approaches for scenario planning and stockpiling strategies?
- What options and strategies could be considered to inform the smallpox MCM stockpiling posture?
- How can the lessons from COVID-19 and mpox inform the U.S. preparedness and readiness posture?

3:45 p.m.   **Scenario Planning and MCM Stockpiling Strategies**
                   HENRY WILLIS, *Moderator, Committee Member*

                   NATHANIEL HUPERT
                   Associate Professor of Population Health Sciences
                   Cornell University Weill Medical College

                   CRYSTAL WATSON
                   Senior Scholar and Associate Professor
                   Johns Hopkins Center for Health Security

                   KEVIN YESKEY
                   Senior Advisor for Emergency Public Health
                   MDB, Inc.

                   SESSION V Wrap-Up and Closing Remarks

4:25 p.m.   **Summary of Day 1 and Closing Remarks**

                   LARRY GOSTIN, *Committee Chair*
                   Distinguished University Professor and O'Neill Chair
                   in Global Health Law
                   O'Neill Institute for National and Global Health Law
                   Georgetown University

4:30 p.m.   **ADJOURN**

PUBLIC WORKSHOP AGENDA (DAY 2)

Friday, December 15, 2023

Purpose
- Discuss how the COVID-19 pandemic and the mpox multi-country outbreak can inform improvements to smallpox readiness and response.
- Explore how recent COVID-19 and mpox public health emergencies have altered assumptions about the U.S. stockpiling, preparedness, and readiness posture.

SESSION VI Day 2 Opening Session

12:30 p.m.   **Welcoming Remarks**
                    LARRY GOSTIN, *Committee Chair*
                    Distinguished University Professor and O'Neill Chair
                    in Global Health Law
                    O'Neill Institute for National and Global Health Law
                    Georgetown University

SESSION VII Synthetic Biology Opportunities and Risks

Objectives: *(1) Hear briefing on advancements in synthetic biology related to smallpox, and (2) examine the opportunities and risks that these advancements pose to preparedness, readiness, and response capabilities and capacities.*

Guiding Questions:
- What is the likelihood for advancements in synthetic biology to develop a poxvirus with pandemic potential?
- How do advancements in synthetic biology alter approaches to preparedness, readiness, and robust public health response to smallpox?
- What opportunities and risks do these advancements pose to preparedness and readiness capabilities and capacities of the United States?

12:35 p.m.   **Synthetic Biology**
                    DREW ENDY, *Moderator, Committee Member*

                    CATHRYN MAYES
                    Senior Biologist
                    Sandia Laboratories

SESSION VIII Lessons Learned and Future Considerations for Smallpox Preparedness and Readiness

Objectives: *Explore how recent COVID-19 and mpox public health emergencies have altered assumptions about preparedness, readiness, and MCMs stockpiling posture for smallpox.*

Guiding Questions:
- How has the 2022 mpox multi-country outbreak altered our assumption about the availability of smallpox medical countermeasures (MCMs) and the ability to meet potential demand?
- How can the lessons from COVID-19 and mpox inform the U.S. stockpiling, preparedness, and readiness posture?
- What additional areas of research and development could be conducted to improve our MCMs?

12:45 p.m.   **Lessons Learned and Future Considerations**
                  GEORGES BENJAMIN, *Moderator, Committee Member*

                  MATTHEW HEPBURN
                  Chief Medical Officer
                  JPEO-CBRND

                  EWA KING
                  Chief Program Officer
                  Association of Public Health Laboratories (APHL)

                  MARCUS PLESCIA
                  Chief Medical Officer
                  Association of State and Territorial Health Officials
                  (ASTHO)

SESSION IX Wrap-Up and Closing Remarks

1:45 p.m.   **Concluding Remarks**
                  LARRY GOSTIN, *Committee Chair*
                  Distinguished University Professor and O'Neill Chair in Global Health Law
                  O'Neill Institute for National and Global Health Law
                  Georgetown University

2:00 p.m.   **ADJOURN**

MEETING 4 AGENDA

Friday, January 12, 2024

Purpose
- Engage in discussion with external subject matter experts on issues related to smallpox medical countermeasures, specifically diagnostics and therapeutics.

SESSION X Presentations and Discussion on Key Issues Related to Smallpox Diagnostics and Therapeutics

Objective: *To hold a discussion with key subject matter experts on key issues related to the study charge.*

2:30 p.m.	**Welcoming Remarks** LARRY GOSTIN, *Committee Chair* Distinguished University Professor and O'Neill Chair in Global Health Law O'Neill Institute for National and Global Health Law Georgetown University
2:35 p.m.	**DoD Presentations and Discussions on Smallpox Diagnostics and Therapeutics** NICOLE DORSEY Director, Advanced Technology Platforms and Clinical Evaluation (ATP) Joint Project Lead, CBRND Enabling Biotechnologies (JPL CBRND EB) MATTHEW CLARK Colonel, U.S. Army Joint Project Manager, CBRN Medical Joint Program Executive Office for Chemical, Biological, Radiological and Nuclear Defense (JPEO-CBRND)
3:15 p.m.	**Presentations and Discussions on Smallpox Diagnostics** GAVIN CLOHERTY Senior Research Fellow, Head of Infectious Disease Research Abbott Molecular Diagnostics

MANOJ GANDHI
Senior Director for Medical and Scientific Affairs
Abbott Molecular Diagnostics

JOHN CONNOR
Associate Professor of Virology, Immunology, and
Microbiology
Boston University

3:45 p.m.   **Q&A with CDC**
CHRISTY HUTSON
Chief, Poxvirus and Rabies Branch
Division of High Consequence Pathogens and
Pathology
U.S. Centers for Disease Control and Prevention
(CDC)

3:55 p.m.   **Wrap-Up and Closing Remarks**
LARRY GOSTIN, *Committee Chair*
Distinguished University Professor and O'Neill Chair
in Global Health Law
O'Neill Institute for National and Global Health Law
Georgetown University

4:00 p.m.   **ADJOURN**

B

Committee and Staff
Biographical Sketches

COMMITTEE MEMBERS

Lawrence Gostin, J.D., L.L.D. (*Chair*), is Distinguished University Professor, the highest academic rank at Georgetown University, where he directs the World Health Organization Collaborating Center on National and Global Health Law and also the O'Neill Institute for National and Global Health Law. He has worked at the intersection of law, national and global health, and ethics and had deep engagement with major novel infectious disease outbreaks, including SARS, Ebola, Zika, influenza H1N1, and COVID-19. In 2016, Gostin received the Adam Yarmolinsky Medal from the National Academies of Sciences, Engineering, and Medicine (the National Academies) for "distinguished service by a Member who, over a significant period of time, has contributed in multiple ways to the mission of the Institute of Medicine." In 2015 the American Public Health Association conferred on him a lifetime achievement award. Professor Gostin has chaired and served on multiple expert National Academies committees and has served on several National Academies boards, including global health, population health, and health sciences policy.

Georges C. Benjamin, M.D., is a well-known health policy leader, practitioner, and administrator. He currently serves as the executive director of the American Public Health Association, the nation's oldest and largest organization of public health professionals. He is also a former secretary of health for the state of Maryland. Dr. Benjamin is a graduate of the Illinois Institute of Technology and the University of Illinois College of Medicine. He is board certified in internal medicine, a master of the American College of Physicians, a fellow of the National Academy of Public Administration, a fellow emeritus of the American College of Emergency Physicians, and a member of the National Academy of Medicine. He serves on several nonprofit boards such as Research!America, the Truth Foundation, and the Reagan-Udall Foundation. He is a former member of the National Infrastructure Advisory Council, a council that advises the president on how best to assure the security of the nation's critical infrastructure.

Nahid Bhadelia, M.D., M.A.L.D., is the founding director of Boston University (BU) Center on Emerging Infectious Diseases. She is a board-certified infectious diseases physician and an associate professor at the BU School of Medicine. She served as the senior policy advisor for global COVID-19 response for the White House COVID-19 Response Team in 2022–2023 as well as the interim testing coordinator on the White House mpox response team. Between 2011 and 2021, Dr. Bhadelia helped develop and then served as the medical director of the Special Pathogens Unit (SPU) at Boston Medical Center, a medical unit designed to care for patients with highly communicable diseases. She was also previously an associate director for BU's maximum containment research program, the National Emerging Infectious Diseases Laboratories. She has provided direct care and helped lead medical and research response to multiple viral hemorrhagic fever outbreaks in East and West Africa. Dr. Bhadelia's research focuses on global health security and pandemic preparedness, including medical countermeasure evaluation and clinical care for emerging infections, diagnostics evaluation and positioning, infection control policy development, and health care worker training. She is a member of the National Academies Forum on Microbial Threats.

Inger Damon, M.D., Ph.D., retired from the U.S. Centers for Disease Control and Prevention (CDC) in September 2022, where her career spanned 23 years of work on deadly diseases and associated preparedness and response efforts. Currently, she continues to hold an adjunct faculty position with Emory University School of Medicine. She is one of the world's experts on orthopoxviruses, including smallpox, an infectious disease that killed millions before it was declared eradicated in 1980 by global surveillance and vaccination campaigns. For over 15 years, Dr. Damon directed CDC's smallpox research program, conducting research to help develop new smallpox diagnostic tests, assess the effectiveness of new vaccines, and create better drugs for treatment. Her expertise leading this global poxvirus activity included programs to look for sources of poxviruses in wildlife, leading CDC's 2003 response to an outbreak of monkeypox in the United States linked to imported exotic pets, and reestablishment of collaborative work on mpox in the Congo Basin. From 2014 to 2022, Dr.

Damon served as the director for the Division of High Consequence Pathogens and Pathology, overseeing the agency's expertise on deadly pathogens such as Ebola, other viral hemorrhagic fever viruses, smallpox, rabies, and anthrax. The division has responsibility for a broad range of bacterial and viral pathogens, myalgic encephalomyelitis/chronic fatigue syndrome, and prion diseases and cross-cutting pathology roles. She served as the incident manager for CDC's response to the Ebola epidemic in West Africa to help direct the agency's national and global fight against Ebola.

Dr. Damon has worked with multiple international organizations. Most recently, she served as rapporteur on the International Health Regulations emergency committee on the multi-country outbreak of mpox and on the standing recommendations committee. She served as a member of the scientific advisory board for Coalition for Epidemic Preparedness Innovations from 2017 to 2023 and has been a member of the World Heath Organization (WHO) Advisory Committee on Variola Virus Research since 2018. Dr. Damon has participated as a work group member with the Advisory Committee on Immunization Practices (ACIP) to review information to contribute to ACIP decision making on orthopoxvirus and mpox vaccination recommendations in the United States. Dr. Damon has participated as a member of U.S. interagency smallpox preparedness efforts in the Public Health Emergency Countermeasure Enterprise (PHEMCE). In October 2023, Dr. Damon joined the WHO R&D Pathogen Prioritization workgroup considering Poxvirus family pathogens. Dr. Damon has been a member of the WHO Scientific Advisory Group on the Origins of Novel Pathogens (SAGO) since its inception. Dr. Damon is a co-inventor on a patent for a poxvirus diagnostic assay. Dr Damon has published, with multiple co-authors and collaborators, over 200 peer reviewed manuscripts, agency documents, or textbook chapters related to research to understand responding to orthopoxviruses and emerging pathogens. Her efforts and work have been recognized both within the U.S. government and externally through multiple awards. Recent recognitions include CDC's Lifetime Scientific Achievement Award in 2022, an honorary doctorate of science from Amherst College in 2016, and the United States Public Health Service Distinguished Service Medal in 2017. Dr. Damon completed a combined M.D.–Ph.D. program at the University of Connecticut Health Center in 1992, and received a B.A., magna cum laude in chemistry from Amherst College in 1984. She trained in internal medicine at the Hospital of the University of Pennsylvania (1992–1995) and completed a fellowship in infectious diseases at the National Institute of Allergy and Infectious Diseases in 1999, where she worked in the laboratory of Dr. Bernard Moss.

Andrew Endy, Ph.D., is a bioengineer at Stanford University who studies and teaches synthetic biology. His goals are civilization-scale flourishing and renewal of liberal democracies. Dr. Endy helped launch new undergraduate majors in bioengineering at both the Massachusetts Institute of Technology and Stanford University and the iGEM—a global genetic-engineering "Olympics" enabling thousands of students annually. His past students lead such companies as Ginkgo Bioworks and Octant. He has financial interests in several synthetic biology companies. Dr. Endy served on the U.S. National Science Advisory Board for Biosecurity (NSABB), the Committee on Science, Technology, and Law (CSTL), the International Union for the Conservation of Nature's Synthetic Biology Task Force, and, briefly, the Pentagon's Defense Innovation Board. He currently serves on the World Health Organization's Advisory Committee on Variola Virus Research, the Defense Science Board's Emerging Biotechnologies Task Force, and the Organization for Economic Co-operation and Development's Synthetic Biology Task Force. He also serves on the boards of the BioBricks, iGEM, and BioBuilder Educational Foundations, public benefit charities advancing open source biotechnologies and bioengineering education. *Esquire* magazine recognized Dr. Drew as one of the 75 most influential people of the 21st century.

Diane E. Griffin, M.D., Ph.D., is University Distinguished Service Professor and former chair of the W. Harry Feinstone Department of Molecular Microbiology and Immunology at Johns Hopkins Bloomberg School of Public Health. Dr. Griffin is a virologist recognized for her work on the pathogenesis of viral infections. She is known particularly for her studies on measles and alphavirus encephalomyelitis which have delineated the role of the immune response in virus clearance, vaccine-induced protection from infection, tissue damage, and immune suppression. She has over 400 publications and has received the Rudolf Virchow Medal from the University of Wurzburg, the Wallace Sterling Award from Stanford University, the FASEB Excellence in Science Award, and the Maxwell Finland Award from the National Foundation for Infectious Diseases. Dr. Griffin graduated from Augustana College with a B.A. in biology and from Stanford University School of Medicine with an M.D. and Ph.D., followed by residency in internal medicine. She was a postdoctoral fellow in virology and infectious diseases at Johns Hopkins University School of Medicine. She has been president of the American Society for Virology and the American Society for Microbiology and is currently vice president of the National Academy of Sciences and U.S. Chair of the U.S.–Japan Cooperative Medical Sciences Program. She serves on vaccine advisory committees for GSK and Tekeda Pharmaceuticals and has received research funding from Merck and Gilead Biosciences in addition to the National Institutes of Health. She is an elected member of the National Academy of Medicine, American Academy of Microbiology, Association of American Physicians, and the American Philosophical Society.

Noreen Hynes, M.D., M.P.H., is currently associate professor at Johns Hopkins University (JHU) Schools of Medicine and Public Health with appointments in infectious diseases (Department of Medicine) and public health (departments of international health, environmental health and engineering, and population/family/reproductive health) and serves as the research director and associate medical director of the Johns Hopkins Hospital Biocontainment Unit. Dr. Hynes spent over 30 years working in the U.S. government including the Peace Corps, Department of State, Department of Health and Human Services (HHS), and the Office of the Vice President of the United States. She has worked both internationally and domestically providing medical care, working with and at state/county/local health departments, teaching (bedside and classroom), and undertaking research (laboratory-based vaccine [Ebola, dengue, COVID-19] and therapeutic randomized clinical trials [COVID-19 ACTT], implementation science [COVID-19], and disease surveillance). Since 1997 she has increasingly focused on high-consequence pathogens, particularly Category A agents, including as a deputy assistant secretary in the Office of Public Health Preparedness and Response (now ASPR), and the director of the Office of Public Health Emergency Medical Countermeasures, now the Biomedical Advanced Research and Development Authority, and she created the Office of Public Health Emergency Countermeasures. In the latter setting, Dr Hynes ran an $8 billion program to develop and acquire medical countermeasures (MCMs) for the Strategic National Stockpile, including smallpox MCMs (live, replicating smallpox vaccine [ACAM2000], live non-replicating smallpox vaccine [MVA-BN/Jynneos], ST-246 [tecovirimat/Tpoxx]), anthrax MCMs, and pandemic influenza MCMs. Dr. Hynes is trained as a physician and has completed a residency in internal medicine and a fellowship in infectious diseases at Harvard's Massachusetts General Hospital, a master of public health at JHU, field epidemiology as an Epidemic Intelligence Service officer at the U.S. Centers for Disease Control and Prevention, and a diploma in tropical medicine and hygiene from the Royal College of Physicians/London School of Tropical Medicine and Hygiene. She has received numerous awards including the HHS Secretary's Award for outstanding Service, the U.S. Public Health Service's Distinguished Service Medal, and the Leadership Program for Women Faculty at JHU. Dr. Hynes has published over 100 journal articles and book chapters.

Richard Kennedy, Ph.D., is a professor of medicine and the co-director of Mayo Clinic's Vaccine Research Group. He has over 150 peer-reviewed publications. He is the deputy editor-in-chief of *Vaccine: X*, an associate editor at *Vaccine*, and an associate editor for *Frontiers in Immunology*. He is a member of the American Association of Immunologists and the American Society for Microbiology. He has served as a reviewer for dozens of National Institutes of Health (NIH) study sections and has participated in numerous national and international review panels. Dr. Kennedy has multiple R01 grants from NIH funding his work on viral vaccine immunology. Dr. Kennedy has also received foundation and industry funding to study adverse events after COVID-19 vaccination and to develop peptide-based vaccines for COVID-19, respectively. His research emphasis is on understanding the factors driving the tremendous diversity in human immune responses to vaccines against viral pathogens, including influenza, measles, mumps, rubella, SARS-CoV-2, smallpox, varicella, and Zika. Dr. Kennedy has authored the smallpox and vaccinia chapter in the textbook *Vaccines*, served as an advisor for the WHO Global Advisory Committee on Vaccine Safety in 2015, wrote the report *Emergency Stockpiling and Future Use of Smallpox Vaccines* for that committee, and served as an external advisor for the WHO Strategic Advisory Group of Experts—Monkeypox Working Group in 2022. Dr. Kennedy is also a member of the Joint Scientific Committee for Phase 1 Clinical Trials for the Queen Mary Hospital (The University of Hong Kong) and Prince of Wales Hospital (The Chinese University of Hong Kong).

Kent Kester, M.D., is currently the vice president of translational medicine at the International AIDS Vaccine Initiative. During a 24-year career in the U.S. Army, he worked extensively in clinical vaccine development and led multiple research platforms at the Walter Reed Army Institute of Research, the Department of Defense's largest and most diverse biomedical research laboratory with a major emphasis on emerging infectious diseases, an institution he later led as its commander. His final military assignment was as the associate dean for clinical research in the School of Medicine at the Uniformed Services University of the Health Sciences (USUHS). During his military service, Dr. Kester was appointed as the lead policy advisor to the U.S. Army Surgeon General both in infectious diseases and in medical research and development. More recently, he served as the head of translational medicine and biomarkers at Sanofi Pasteur. Dr. Kester holds an undergraduate degree from Bucknell University and an M.D. from Jefferson Medical College; he completed his internship and residency in internal medicine at the University of Maryland and a research fellowship in infectious diseases at the Walter Reed Army Medical Center. Currently a member of the Department of Veterans Affairs (VA) Health Services Research and Development Service Merit Review Board, the National Academy Standing Committee on Emerging Infectious Diseases and 21st Century Health Threats, and the Coalition for Epidemic Preparedness Initiative scientific advisory committee, he previously chaired the steering committee of the National Institute of Allergy and Infectious Diseases (NIAID)/USUHS Infectious Disease Clinical Research Program, and he has served as a member of the Presidential Advisory Council on Combating Antibiotic-Resistant Bacteria, the U.S. Food and Drug Administration's Vaccines and Related Biologics Products Advisory

Committee, the NIAID advisory council, and the board of scientific counselors for the Office of Infectious Diseases at the U.S. Centers for Disease Control and Prevention. He is the vice chair of the National Academy of Medicine Forum on Microbial Threats. Board-certified in both internal medicine and infectious diseases, Dr. Kester holds faculty appointments at USUHS and the University of Maryland and is a fellow of the American College of Physicians, the Royal College of Physicians of Edinburgh, the Infectious Disease Society of America, and the American Society of Tropical Medicine and Hygiene. He is a member of the clinical faculty at the University of Maryland Shock Trauma Center in Baltimore and the Wilkes-Barre VA Medical Center in Wilkes-Barre, Pennsylvania. He has ownership of (former employee) stock in a pharmaceutical company that does not work in the area of smallpox and related vaccines.

Anne Rimoin, Ph.D., M.P.H., is a professor of epidemiology and the Gordon-Levin Endowed Chair in Infectious Diseases and Public Health at the University of California, Los Angeles (UCLA) Fielding School of Public Health. She is the director of the Center for Global and Immigrant Health and the director and founder of the UCLA-DRC Health Research and Training Program. She is a globally recognized expert on infectious diseases, global health, disease surveillance systems, and vaccination. Dr. Rimoin has been leading studies of emerging and vaccine preventable diseases for more than two decades. Her work has contributed to the fundamental understanding of the epidemiology of human mpox, long-term immunity to Ebola virus in survivors, and durability of immune response to Ebola virus vaccines in health workers. Her current research portfolio includes studies of Congo Crimean hemorrhagic fever, COVID-19, Ebola virus, Nipahvirus, Marburg, mpox, and vaccine-preventable diseases of childhood. She is considered one of the world's leading subject matter experts on the epidemiology of mpox and participated on the World Health Organization (WHO) International Health Regulations Emergency Committee on the multi-country outbreak of mpox and the WHO Strategic Advisory Group of Experts on Immunization Working Group on Smallpox and Mpox. She has been recognized for her achievements in the fields of epidemiology and global health with the Middlebury College Alumni Achievement Award (2017), induction as a fellow of the American Society of Tropical Medicine and Hygiene (2019), and the Johns Hopkins Alumni Association Global Achievement Award (2021). Dr. Rimoin earned her B.A. at Middlebury College, M.P.H. at UCLA, and Ph.D. at Johns Hopkins University. She started her career in global public health as a Peace Corps volunteer in Benin, West Africa, in the Guinea Worm Eradication Program.

Oyewale Tomori, D.V.M., Ph.D., is a past president of the Nigerian Academy of Science with experience in virology, disease prevention, and control. He was a researcher at the University of Ibadan from 1971 to 1994.

He later served as the pioneer vice chancellor of the Redeemer's University in Nigeria from 2004 to 2011. From 1994 to 2004, he was the virologist for the WHO-AFRO, establishing the African Regional Polio Laboratory Network. In 1981, he was recognized by the U.S. Centers for Disease Control and Prevention for contributions to Lassa fever research. In 2002, he received the Nigerian National Order of Merit, the country's highest award for academic and intellectual attainment and national development. Dr. Tomori has served or continues to serve on numerous advisory committees, at national and global levels, including (national) Lassa Fever Steering Committee, Laboratory Technical Working Group, Expert Group on Polio Eradication and Routine Immunization, and Advisory Committee on COVID-19 Response, and (international) World Health Organization (WHO) SAGE, WHO-AFRO Polio Certification Committee, WHO Yellow Fever Disease Committee, WHO TAG on COVID-19 Vaccine Composition, GAVI Board, U.S. National Academies of Sciences, Engineering, and Medicine Global Health Risk Framework Commission, and WHO-AFRO Laboratory Planning and Quality Monitoring Adviser. He is a member of U.S. National Academy of Medicine. He has authored or co-authored over 160 scientific publications. Dr. Tomori currently serves as a non-executive chair of the board of directors of BioVaccines Nigeria Limited (BVNL), a joint special purpose vehicle company set up between the Federal Government of Nigeria (FGN) and the May and Baker Company, a private pharmaceutical company, to manufacture locally vaccines for childhood vaccinations in Nigeria. The board provides guidance and policy oversight to the Management of BVNL. It is a non-remunerative position. Dr. Tomori is one of the three representatives of the FGN in the BVNL Board.

Henry Willis, Ph.D., is a senior policy researcher at the RAND Corporation and a professor of policy analysis at the Pardee RAND Graduate School. He previously served as deputy director of the RAND Homeland Security Division and director of the division's Strategy, Policy, and Operations Program and Infrastructure, Immigration, and Security Operations Program. Dr. Willis is a recognized expert in risk analysis and management. Recent work analyzes biosecurity risks and biodefense capabilities; food, energy, and water security; climate and natural disaster risks; critical infrastructure resilience; national preparedness to chemical, biological, nuclear, and radiological attacks; and prevention of global catastrophic and existential risk. Through his work he testified before Congress; served on several committees of the National Academies of Sciences, Engineering, and Medicine; advised government agencies across the United States, Europe, Australia, and the United Arab Emirates; and published dozens of journal articles, reports, and op-eds on applying risk analysis to homeland security policy. Dr. Willis is a member of the Council on Foreign Relations and serves on the science and governance committees of the Society for Risk Analysis. His work in homeland security policy evolved from his work on program evaluation at the White House Office of Management and Budget and infrastructure design as a water and wastewater engineer. He earned his Ph.D. in engineering and public policy at Carnegie Mellon University, M.S. in environmental engineering from the University of Cincinnati, and B.A. in chemistry from the University of Pennsylvania.

Matthew Wynia, M.D., M.P.H., is board certified in internal medicine and infectious diseases, with additional training in public health and health services research. He led the Institute for Ethics at the American Medical Association for 15 years and founded its Center for Patient Safety before moving in 2015 to become the director of the University of Colorado (CU) Center for Bioethics and Humanities (CBH). The CBH is involved in the education for every health professions student at CU, facilitates clinical ethics case consultation for hospitals on the Anschutz Medical Campus, and carries out a research agenda to better understand the complex ethical challenges facing medicine and society. The center also runs the annual Aspen Ethical Leadership Program and several major community engagement programs, including the annual Holocaust Genocide Contemporary Bioethics program and the Hard Call® podcast series. Dr. Wynia has led national projects on issues including public health and disaster ethics; ethics and quality improvement; communication, team-based care and engaging patients as members of the team; and medicine and the Holocaust. He has delivered more than two dozen named lectures and visiting professorships and is the author of more than 160 published articles, co-editor of several books, and co-author of a book on fairness in health care benefit design. He is a fellow of the Hastings Center, past president of the American Society for Bioethics and Humanities, and past chair of the Ethics Forum of the American Public Health Association and the Ethics Committee of the Society for General Internal Medicine.

Zhilong Yang, Ph.D., is an associate professor in the Department of Veterinary Pathobiology, School of Veterinary Medicine and Biomedical Sciences at Texas A&M University. He has been working on large DNA viruses for over 21 years, including over 15 years on poxviruses. His current research focuses on understanding how poxviruses replicate in their infected host cells, antiviral discovery, and poxvirus utility development. He is a member of American Society for Virology as well as a member of American Society for Microbiology. He obtained his B.S. and M.S. degrees from Nankai University and his Ph.D. degree from University of Nebraska–Lincoln, and he received postdoc training in the Laboratory of Viral Diseases at the National Institute of Allergy and Infectious Diseases.

STAFF AND CONSULTANT BIOS

Lisa Brown, M.P.H. (*Study Director*), is a senior program officer on the Board on Health Sciences Policy at the National Academies of Sciences, Engineering, and Medicine (the National Academies) and develops and manages projects at the National Academies related to solving the nation's most pressing health security issues. She currently serves as a director for the Standing Committee on Emerging Infectious Diseases and 21st Century Health Threats and the Forum on Medical and Public Health Preparedness for Disasters and Emergencies. She has directed several projects, including the Committee on Equitable Allocation of Vaccine for the Novel Coronavirus, the Committee on Data Needs to Monitor Evolution of SARS-CoV-2, the Committee on Evidence-Based Practices for Public Health Emergency Preparedness and Response, and the Committee on Strengthening the Disaster Resilience of Academic Research Communities. Prior to the National Academies, Ms. Brown served as senior program analyst for public health preparedness and environment health at the National Association of County and City Health Officials (NACCHO). In this capacity, Ms. Brown served as project lead for medical countermeasures and the Strategic National Stockpile, researched radiation preparedness issues, and was involved in high-level U.S. Centers for Disease Control and Prevention initiatives for the development of clinical guidance for smallpox, anthrax, and botulism countermeasures in a mass casualty event. In 2015, she was selected as a fellow in the Emerging Leaders in Biosecurity Initiative at the Center for Health Security, a highly competitive program to prepare the next generation of leaders in the field of biosecurity. Prior to her work at NACCHO, Ms. Brown worked as an Environmental Public Health Scientist at Public Health England (PHE) in London, England. While at PHE, she focused on climate change, the recovery process following disasters, and the impact of droughts and floods on emerging infectious diseases. She received her master of public health from King's College London in 2012 and her bachelor of science in biology from The University of Findlay in 2010.

Shalini Singaravelu, M.Sc., is a program officer at the National Academies of Sciences, Engineering, and Medicine with the Board on Health Sciences Policy, where she supports the Standing Committee on Emerging Infectious Diseases and 21st Century Health Threats and the Forum on Medical and Public Health Preparedness for Disasters and Emergencies. Before joining the National Academies, Ms. Singaravelu managed a portfolio of digital health tools as a program manager at IBM. From 2015 to 2019, she was a consultant for the World Health Organization Health Emergencies Programme in Geneva. In this role, she supported preparedness and response to emerging infectious disease epidemics with a focus on operational data systems, risk communication, and community engagement. Prior to this, she worked on psychosocial support programming for HIV-affected or-phans and vulnerable children in South Africa. Ms. Singaravelu was a 2022 Emerging Leaders in Biosecurity Initiative (ELBI) Fellow with the Johns Hopkins Center for Health Security. She has a graduate certificate in risk sciences and public policy from Johns Hopkins Bloomberg School of Public Health (2021), where she is currently a Dr.P.H. candidate in environmental health and health security. She received her M.Sc. in global mental health from the London School of Hygiene and Tropical Medicine (2014) and a B.A. in anthropology from Union College (2012).

Matthew Masiello, M.P.H., is an associate program officer on the Board on Health Sciences Policy at the National Academies of Sciences, Engineer-ing, and Medicine where he supports projects that focus on health security and public health emergency preparedness and response. He completed his M.P.H. in May 2021 at Emory University Rollins School of Public Health, where he focused on disaster epidemiology and COVID-19 vaccine uptake. His thesis measured COVID-19 vaccine intent among the Emory student body and captured predictors for vaccine uptake and hesitancy. While completing his M.P.H., Mr. Masiello interned at the Council for State and Territorial Epidemiologists where he supported the Tribal Epidemiology Subcommittee and the Epidemiological Capacity Assessment. Prior to his M.P.H. program, Mr. Masiello spent 3 years at the National Academies supporting four consensus studies across the Health and Medicine Division. He earned his B.A. at American University in May 2016.

Margaret McCarthy, M.Sc., is a research associate with the International Networks and Cooperation Theme within the Policy and Global Affairs Division. She previously worked with the Board on Health Sciences Policy within the Health and Medicine Division for the last 2.5 years on projects related to health security and pandemic preparedness. Before joining the National Academies, Ms. McCarthy worked at Brigham and Women's Hospital in the Division of Infectious Diseases. She graduated from Ameri-can University with a B.A. in international studies and a master's degree in global health and development from University College London. She is currently pursuing an online, part-time master's degree in global security from King's College London.

Claire Biffl, B.A., is a research associate working on the Forum on Microbial Threats within the Board on Global Health at the National Academies. Her recent work has focused on pandemic preparedness, antimicrobial resistance, and arboviral threats. She graduated with High Honors from Emory University in 2020 after earning a B.A. in an-thropology and a minor in political science. Her senior thesis was an

ethnographic study of gerontological topics as observed in an independent senior living facility in Georgia.

Rayane Silva-Curran is a senior program assistant on the Board on Health
Sciences Policy, with the Forum on Medical and Public Health Preparedness for Disasters and Emergencies. Before joining the National Academies, Ms. Silva-Curran worked as a COVID-19 contact tracer for the
Fairfax County Health Department. She received her B.S. in community
health with a concentration in global health from George Mason University. She also holds a B.S. in biology from the Universidade Estadual de
Goias (Brazil).

Kavita Berger, Ph.D., is the director of the Board on Life Sciences and co-
director of the Board on Animal Health Sciences, Conservation, and Research of the National Academies of Sciences, Engineering, and Medicine.
She is a life scientist with extensive experience in the addressing a diversity
of technical, policy, national security, and societal issues associated with the
life sciences and biotechnology. Dr. Berger leads and oversees the Board on
Life Sciences' work across a variety of life science areas, including basic, applied, and emerging life sciences research; biotechnology research and convergence; bioeconomy-related research and development; biosecurity and
biodefense; ecology and biodiversity; and integrated human, animal, plant,
and ecological health. Prior to joining the National Academies, Dr. Berger
was a principal scientist at Gryphon Scientific. There she led numerous projects involving biotechnology landscape analyses, biosecurity and biodefense
policy, risk and benefits of life science research and technologies, and international bioengagement. Dr. Berger was responsible for several biosecurity
and biodefense initiatives at the American Association for the Advancement
of Science, including a meeting series on topics ranging from health security
to preventing biological weapons. Dr. Berger has served on two National
Research Council committees related to cooperative biological engagement,
on the board of directors for the nongovernmental Global Health Security
Agenda Consortium, and as a subject matter expert for various government
and nongovernmental organizations. A list of Dr. Berger's publications is
accessible through her MyNCBI bibliography. Dr. Berger has a Ph.D. in
genetics and molecular biology from Emory University and conducted preclinical research on HIV and smallpox vaccines.

Julie Pavlin, M.D., Ph.D., M.P.H., is the director of the Board on Global
Health at the National Academies of Sciences, Engineering, and Medicine
where she coordinates analyses of health developments beyond U.S. borders
and areas of international health investment that promote global well-
being, security, and economic development. Prior to this position, she was

a research area director at the Infectious Disease Clinical Research Program and the deputy director of the Armed Forces Health Surveillance Center. She is a retired Colonel in the U.S. Army with previous assignments including the Armed Forces Research Institute of Medical Sciences in Bangkok, Thailand; the Walter Reed Army Institute of Research; and the U.S. Army Medical Research Institute for Infectious Diseases. She concentrated most of her time with the Department of Defense in the design of real-time disease surveillance systems and was a co-founder of the International Society for Disease Surveillance. Dr. Pavlin received her A.B. from Cornell University, M.D. from Loyola University, M.P.H. from Harvard University, and Ph.D. in emerging infectious diseases at the Uniformed Services University.

Clare Stroud, Ph.D., is the senior board director for the Board on Health Sciences Policy at the National Academies of Sciences, Engineering, and Medicine. In this capacity, she oversees a program of activities aimed at fostering the basic biomedical and clinical research enterprises; addressing the ethical, legal, and social contexts of scientific and technologic advances related to health; and strengthening the preparedness, resilience, and sustainability of communities. Previously, she served as director of the National Academies' Forum on Neuroscience and Nervous System Disorders, which brings together leaders from government, academia, industry, and nonprofit organizations to discuss key challenges and emerging issues in neuroscience research, development of therapies for nervous system disorders, and related ethical and societal issues. She also led consensus studies and contributed to projects on topics such as pain management, medications for opioid use disorder, traumatic brain injury, preventing cognitive decline and dementia, supporting persons living with dementia and their caregivers, the health and well-being of young adults, and disaster preparedness and response. Dr. Stroud first joined the National Academies as a Mirzayan Science and Technology Policy Graduate Fellow. She has also been an associate at AmericaSpeaks, a nonprofit organization that engaged citizens in decision making on important public policy issues. Dr. Stroud received her Ph.D. from the University of Maryland, College Park, with research focused on the cognitive neuroscience of language, and her bachelor's degree from Queen's University in Canada.

Ellen P. Carlin, D.V.M., is a veterinarian and policy expert who specializes in emerging infectious disease prevention and preparedness. She is the owner of Parapet Science & Policy Consulting, providing research and writing support for animal and public health projects and initiatives. She supports the implementation of infectious disease research projects in the United States and abroad, analysis and publication of results, and development of policy priorities to address the findings. Her scientific and lay writing has appeared in a variety of platforms read by scientists and by policy makers and their staff, including the *Journal of the American Veterinary Medical Association*, *The Washington Post*, and *The Hill*. Most recently, she co-authored the book *Catastrophic Incentives: Why Our Approaches to Disasters Keep Falling Short* (Columbia University Press, 2023). Dr. Carlin is also a lecturer at the Cornell University College of Veterinary Medicine, where she teaches the next generation of scientists and policy professionals about the role of the federal government in animal health. In 2013 she completed a fellowship at the U.S. Food and Drug Administration Center for Veterinary Medicine. From 2007 to 2013, she staffed the Ranking Member and then Chairman of the House Committee on Homeland Security, where she covered medical preparedness, biodefense, and science and technology. She maintains her license to practice veterinary medicine and has worked or volunteered as a small animal clinical veterinarian to serve her interests in animal welfare, public health, and parasitology. She received a bachelor of science in biology from the College of Mount Saint Vincent and a doctorate in veterinary medicine from the Cornell College of Veterinary Medicine.